Lecture Notes in Computer Science 16254

The series Lecture Notes in Computer Science (LNCS), including its subseries Lecture Notes in Artificial Intelligence (LNAI) and Lecture Notes in Bioinformatics (LNBI), has established itself as a medium for the publication of new developments in computer science and information technology research, teaching, and education.

LNCS enjoys close cooperation with the computer science R & D community, the series counts many renowned academics among its volume editors and paper authors, and collaborates with prestigious societies. Its mission is to serve this international community by providing an invaluable service, mainly focused on the publication of conference and workshop proceedings and postproceedings. LNCS commenced publication in 1973.

Junyu Chen · Aaron Carass · Mattias Heinrich ·
Reuben Dorent
Editors

Medical
Image Registration

International Challenge, Learn2Reg 2025
Held in Conjunction with MICCAI 2025
Daejeon, South Korea, September 27–October 4, 2025
Proceedings

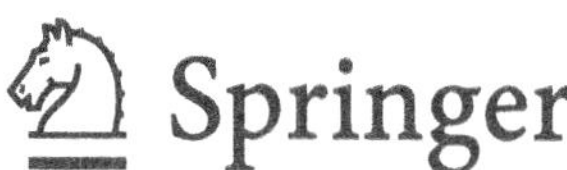

Editors
Junyu Chen
Johns Hopkins University
Baltimore, MD, USA

Aaron Carass
Johns Hopkins University
Baltimore, MD, USA

Mattias Heinrich
University of Lübeck
Lübeck, Germany

Reuben Dorent
Inria-Paris
Paris, France

ISSN 0302-9743 ISSN 1611-3349 (electronic)
Lecture Notes in Computer Science
ISBN 978-3-032-25168-8 ISBN 978-3-032-25169-5 (eBook)
https://doi.org/10.1007/978-3-032-25169-5

This Springer imprint is published by the registered company Springer Nature Switzerland AG
The registered company address is: Gewerbestrasse 11, 6330 Cham, Switzerland

Preface

It is our pleasure to present the proceedings of the 2025 edition of the Learn2Reg Challenge, held in Daejeon, South Korea in conjunction with the 28th International Conference on Medical Image Computing and Computer Assisted Intervention (MICCAI 2025), on September 27th 2025. The Challenge was organized as a collaboration between Johns Hopkins University (Junyu Chen, Aaron Carass, Harrison Bai, & Shuwen Wei), Vanderbilt University (Yihao Liu), University of Lübeck (Mattias P. Heinrich), Inria-Paris (Reuben Dorent & Olivier Colliot), and Harvard University (William M. Well III, Tina Kapur, & Alexandra Golby).

Since 2020 Learn2Reg has been the premier international forum for the presentation of cutting-edge advancements in biomedical image registration. The tasks that constitute each year's Challenge go beyond the boundary of what is currently achievable in the field.

Learn2Reg 2025 had two principle tasks: 1) ReMIND2Reg and 2) LUMIR. The ReMIND2Reg Task was to register multi-parametric pre-operative magnetic resonance images (MRI) and intra-operative 3D ultrasound (US) images. The task was specifically interested in the challenging problem of pre-operative to post-resection registration, requiring the estimation of large deformations and tissue resections. The LUMIR Task was focused on training deep learning registration methods on human brain MRIs, with the evaluation on zero-shot tasks that involve substantial domain shifts. The domain shifts included high-field MRI, pathological brains, alternate MRI contrasts, and non-human brain MRIs.

Both tasks received submissions from twenty-five teams, resulting in thirty-eight unique entries across the two tasks, with repeated submissions excluded from this count. All participating methods are recorded on our live leaderboard. Based on performance on the public validation leaderboard, thirteen entries across the two tasks were invited to submit papers describing the proposed methods. All thirteen invited papers were sent for peer review. The review process was single blind and submissions received two reviews each on average, with reviewers aware of author identities and authors unaware of reviewer identities. Of these thirteen papers, eleven were accepted. Following the subsequent withdrawal of one accepted paper, the final proceedings include ten papers. We are deeply grateful to the reviewers and participating teams for their efforts and commitment to a successful program. We would also like to acknowledge the support of Grand-challenge.org, which has been the online home of the Learn2Reg community since 2020. Without their support and computing services, it would be impossible to host Learn2Reg each year.

The scientific program presented in Daejeon included 10 speakers and multiple poster presentations. We were also fortunate to have Mirabela Rusu from Stanford University present a keynote titled *"Are we there yet?" in multimodal registration?* The prize for the best-performing method on the ReMIND2Reg Task was awarded to Jiazheng Wang

(Hunan University, China), and the LUMIR Task prize went to Hengjie Liu (University of California, San Francisco, USA).

We were honored to organize Learn2Reg 2025 and present the exciting collection of scientific contributions included in these proceedings. Learn2Reg continues to be the premier venue for technological advancements in biomedical image registration and we look forward to Learn2Reg 2026 as the next exciting edition of this wonderful series.

September 2025

Junyu Chen
Aaron Carass
Harrison Bai
Shuwen Wei
Yihao Liu
Mattias Heinrich
Reuben Dorent
Olivier Colliot
William M. Well III
Tina Kapur
Alexandra Golby

Organization

Program Committee Chairs

Junyu Chen	Johns Hopkins University, USA
Aaron Carass	Johns Hopkins University, USA
Harrison Bai	Johns Hopkins University, USA
Shuwen Wei	Johns Hopkins University, USA
Yihao Liu	Vanderbilt University, USA
Mattias P. Heinrich	University of Lübeck, Germany
Reuben Dorent	Inria-Paris, France
Olivier Colliot	Inria-Paris, France
William M. Well III	Harvard University, USA
Tina Kapur	Harvard University, USA
Alexandra Golby	Harvard University, USA

Reviewers

Junyu Chen
Aaron Carass
Hugues Roy
Lianrui Zuo
Reuben Dorent
Shuwen Wei
Zhangxing Bian
Yihao Liu

Contents

ReMIND2Reg

Lumir

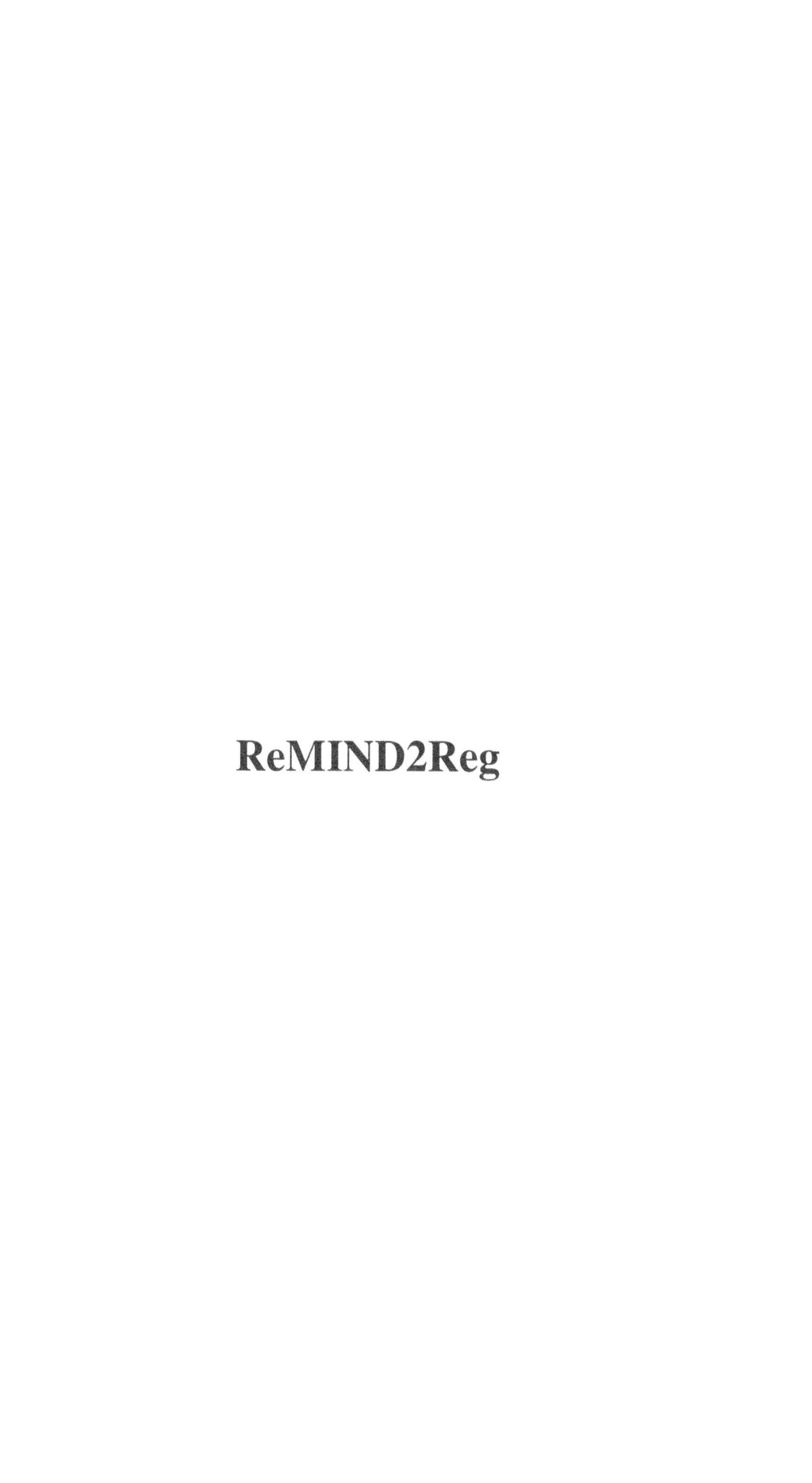

ReMIND2Reg

Unsupervised MR-US Multimodal Image Registration with Multilevel Correlation Pyramidal Optimization

Jiazheng Wang[1,2], Zeyu Liu[1,2], Min Liu[1,2(✉)], Xiang Chen[1,2], Xinyao Yu[3], Yaonan Wang[1,2], and Hang Zhang[4]

[1] School of Artificial Intelligence and Robotics, Hunan University, Changsha, Hunan, China
{wjiazheng,liuzeyulzy,xiangc,yaonan}@hnu.edu.cn
[2] National Engineering Research Center of Robot Visual Perception and Control Technology, Hunan University, Changsha, Hunan, China
liu_min@hnu.edu.cn
[3] National University of Singapore, Singapore, Singapore
xinyao.yu@u.nus.edu
[4] Cornell University, Ithaca, USA
hz459@cornell.edu

Abstract. Surgical navigation based on multimodal image registration has played a significant role in providing intraoperative guidance to surgeons by showing the relative position of the target area to critical anatomical structures during surgery. However, due to the differences between multimodal images and intraoperative image deformation caused by tissue displacement and removal during the surgery, effective registration of preoperative and intraoperative multimodal images faces significant challenges. To address the multimodal image registration challenges in Learn2Reg 2025, an unsupervised multimodal medical image registration method based on Multilevel Correlation Pyramidal Optimization (MCPO) is designed to solve these problems. First, the features of each modality are extracted based on the modality independent neighborhood descriptor, and the multimodal images is mapped to the feature space. Second, a multilevel pyramidal fusion optimization mechanism is designed to achieve global optimization and local detail complementation of the displacement field through dense correlation analysis and weight-balanced coupled convex optimization for input features at different scales. Our method focuses on the ReMIND2Reg task in Learn2Reg 2025. Based on the results, our method achieved the first place in the validation phase and test phase of ReMIND2Reg. The MCPO is also validated on the Resect dataset, achieving an average TRE of 1.798 mm. This demonstrates the broad applicability of our method in preoperative-to-intraoperative image registration. The code is available at https://github.com/wjiazheng/MCPO.

Keywords: Multimodal Medical Image Registration · Convex Optimization · Pyramidal Fusion

J. Chen et al. (Eds.): Learn2Reg 2025, LNCS 16254, pp. 3–11, 2026.
https://doi.org/10.1007/978-3-032-25169-5_1

1 Introduction

Medical image registration has been an important topic in the field of medical image analysis, and many significant methods [2–4,7] have driven the development of medical image registration tasks. Deep learning-based medical image registration methods [6] generally involve long and complex learning processes, and often struggle to achieve accurate estimation for multimodal, large-deformation data and general usability for extensive tasks. The Learn2Reg 2025 sub-challenge, ReMIND2Reg [1], is a multimodal medical image registration task oriented to preoperative Magnetic Resonance Imaging (MRI) and intraoperative ultrasound (US), which is characterized as unlabeled, large deformation, and low feature distinctness. Aiming at the above characteristics, inspired by [8,9], an unsupervised multimodal medical image registration method based on Multilevel Correlation Pyramidal Optimization (MCPO) has been proposed, which can quickly achieve effective MR-US multimodal image registration using only a small number of learning and optimization procedures.

2 Methodology

The proposed MCPO method is based on VoxelOpt [5] and ConvexAdam [10] with a series of improvements, which include (1) Introducing a weight-balancing term on coupled convex optimization to achieve smoother deformation optimization. (2) A multilevel pyramidal fusion optimization mechanism is designed to achieve coarse-to-fine representation of the dense displacement field by performing affine transformation and fusing convex optimization results across different scales. (3) Finally, fine-tuning of the rigid displacement field is achieved through an optional Adam instance optimization.

The overall flow of the proposed MCPO method is shown in Fig. 1. The moving image and the fixed image are inputted and then the modal-independent features of the images are first obtained by Mind-SSC Feature Extractor [9]. The Mind-SSC feature extractor exploits the self-similarity of the partial area in the image to extract the unique structural information of the local neighborhood, which results in a highly consistent structural representation across modalities.

Inspired by VoxelOpt [5], the acquired features are subsequently downsampled by average pooling operations at different times n ($n = 3, 4, 5, 6$) to obtain features in different scales F_n as inputs for the multilevel pyramidal fusion optimization mechanism. For each level, the acquired input features F_n are first fed into the dense correlation layer to compute the sum-of-squared-differences (SSD) cost volume and the initial optimal displacements for each voxel. The large search space allows us to make an initial capture of the displacement for each voxel, even though some voxel points may have large deformations. The output of the dense correlation layer is alternately optimized for similarity and smoothness by iterations in the weight-balanced coupled convex optimization layer, and then the iterative optimization results are averaged to achieve global regularization with weight balancing. After that, an inverse consistency constraint layer [12] is

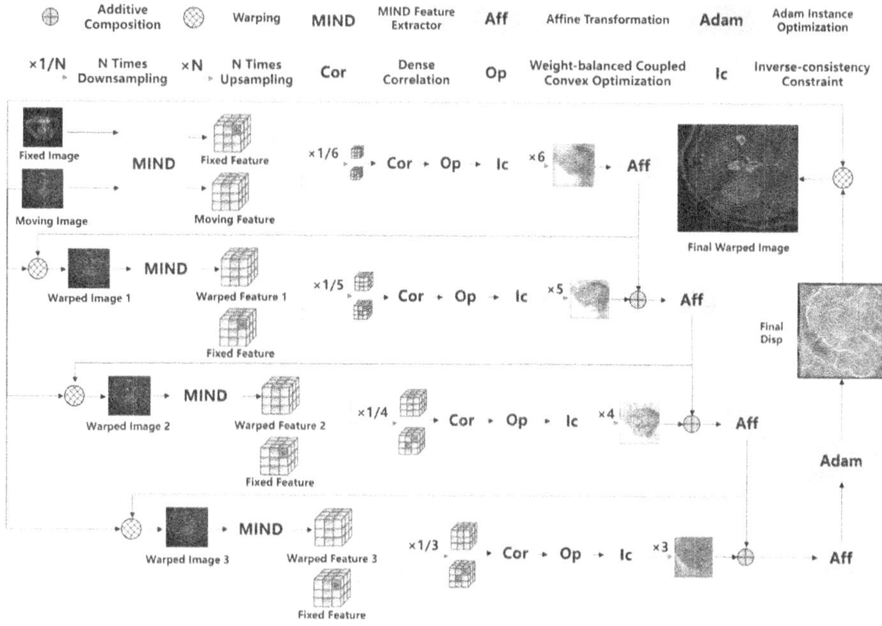

Fig. 1. The overall flow of the proposed MCPO method.

introduced to minimize the difference between the forward and backward transformations to avoid unrealistic deformations, obtaining the initial displacement field of each level. Subsequently, an affine transformation matrix is computed via least-squares fitting to the initial displacement field, yielding a rigid displacement field at each level. The dense displacement field is constructed in a coarse-to-fine manner through additive composition of the rigid displacement field with the subsequent-level field. After completing the additive composition of displacement fields at each level, the final rigid displacement field is obtained.

Furthermore, an optional Adam instance optimization [8] is applied to the final rigid displacement field to further refine the field. In addition to the regularization loss and the Mind loss used in the original Adam instance optimization, we also introduce a stochastic patch-based mutual information loss. Due to the low information density in ultrasound images, the traditional mutual information loss, which relies on global image computations, fails to perform effectively in this task. Therefore, the stochastic patch-based mutual information loss refines the displacement field by randomly sampling informative local patches and comparing their mutual information, thereby leveraging similarities among effective features. Depending on whether Adam instance optimization is employed, two variants of the method are proposed: **MCPO-rigid** and **MCPO-deform**. Their performance is experimentally evaluated and analyzed in the subsequent section.

3 Experiments and Results

Our method focuses on the ReMIND2Reg sub-challenge in Learn2Reg 2025, and to verify the generality of the method, we also tested it on the Resect dataset.

3.1 Dataset

ReMIND2Reg Sub-challenge. The dataset of ReMIND2Reg sub-challenge is a pre-processed subset of the ReMIND dataset [13], which contains pre- and intra-operative data collected on consecutive patients who were surgically treated with image-guided tumor resection between 2018 and 2024. The goal of the ReMIND2Reg sub-challenge is to register pre-operative MRI from multiple modalities (including ceT1 and T2) and intra-operative 3D ultrasound images. Common pre-processing to the same voxel resolution ($0.5 \times 0.5 \times 0.5$ mm) and spatial dimension ($256 \times 256 \times 256$) is performed on all the images. The training set has 99 patients with 99 3D ultrasound images, 93 ceT1 images and 62 T2 images, and the validation set contains 5 patients with 5 images for each modality. The test set is unseen for the participants.

Resect Dataset. The Resect dataset [15] comprises intraoperative ultrasound images and preoperative MRI images from 23 patients with low-grade gliomas. It includes 23 ceT1 MRI scans and 23 FLAIR MRI scans as the moving images. Annotation data for validation are also provided, with each image having dimensions of $256 \times 256 \times 288$ voxels. The patient cohort was selected without significant bias, encompassing tumors located in diverse brain regions, which ensures commendable representativeness and diversity. This dataset serves as an effective resource for validating the performance of different methods.

3.2 Implementation Details

For MCPO-rigid, the radius and dilation of the Mind-SSC feature extractor are fixed to 1 and 2, respectively, and the displacement range of the discretised search space is set to 4. For MCPO-deform, the radius and dilation of the Mind-SSC feature extractor are fixed to 3 and 3, respectively, and the displacement range of the discretised search space is set to 6. For the Adam instance optimization in MCPO-deform, the number of iterations is set to 20, the smooth convolution kernel is set to 5, the weight of the stochastic patch-based mutual information loss is set to 100, and the rest of the parameters are referred to the original settings [10]. These are the parameters that deliver optimal performance with limited runtime determined through multiple experiments.

We employed ConvexAdam [10] with affine transformation, NiftyReg [11], and MCBO [16] as the baseline methods. The evaluation of registration performance in our paper is based on Target Registration Error (TRE), which is defined as the Euclidean distance between corresponding landmarks in the fixed image and the warped moving image. All experiments were conducted using PyTorch, with the instance optimization performed on a single NVIDIA RTX 3090 GPU.

3.3 Experimental Results

Validation Phase of ReMIND2Reg Sub-challenge. The experimental results are shown in Table 1. The visualization of the multimodal image registration for this task is shown in Fig. 2. On the validation set of the ReMIND2Reg Sub-challenge, MCPO-rigid demonstrated optimal performance, achieving a TRE of 1.790 ± 0.536 mm. Although the overall result of MCPO-deform was moderate due to suboptimal performance on a specific case, it remained comparable to baseline methods and marginally outperformed NiftyReg.

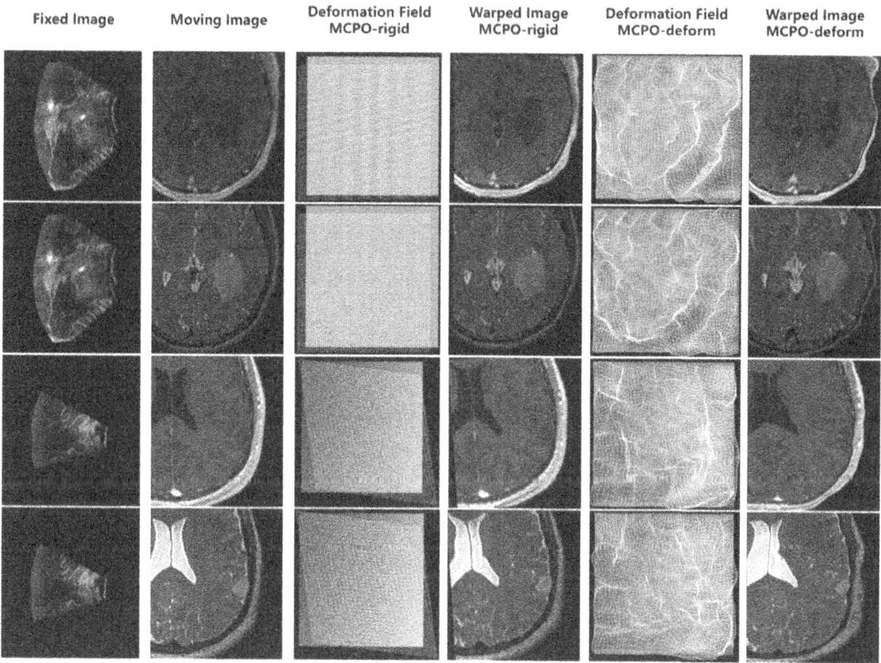

Fig. 2. Visualization results of ReMIND2Reg sub-challenge in Learn2Reg 2025.

Resect Dataset. Since the ReMIND2Reg Sub-challenge includes only five patients (ten cases) with annotation information as the validation set with all exhibiting relatively small deformations, validation based solely on this dataset may lead to potential overfitting to a limited number of similar data, making it difficult to comprehensively evaluate the performance of the methods. Therefore, we conducted additional experiments on the Resect dataset, with results presented in Table 2. On this more diverse dataset, MCPO-deform achieved superior average TRE of 1.798 ± 1.301 mm, while other methods often failed to handle cases with large deformations effectively. As illustrated in Fig. 3, which shows a case from

Table 1. Results of ReMIND2Reg sub-challenge in Learn2Reg 2025.

Methods	TRE(mm)
Initial	3.746 ± 0.639
ConvexAdam-Rigid	2.609 ± 1.217
NiftyReg	2.807 ± 1.228
MCBO	2.367 ± 0.638
MCPO-rigid	**1.790 ± 0.536**
MCPO-deform	2.766 ± 1.001

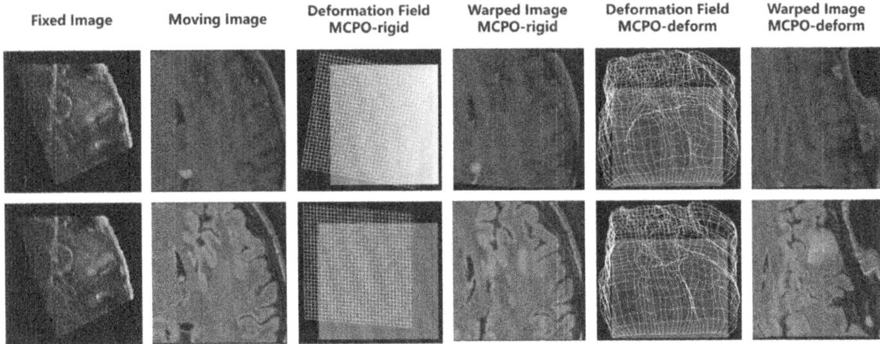

Fig. 3. Visualization results of a large deformation case in the Resect dataset using MCPO-deform.

the Resect dataset with an initial deformation of 19.731 mm, MCPO-deform successfully aligned key anatomical regions between the fixed and warped images. For this case, MCPO-deform achieved registration errors of 1.136 mm (FLAIR to ultrasound) and 1.368 mm (ceT1 to ultrasound). In comparison, MCPO-rigid only reached 13.313 mm and 16.195 mm, respectively. The visualization result for this case is shown in Fig. 4. Considering these results, we ultimately sub-

Table 2. Results of methods in Resect dataset.

Methods	TRE (mm)
Initial	5.374 ± 4.173
ConvexAdam-Rigid	2.673 ± 1.474
NiftyReg	2.635 ± 3.009
MCBO	3.785 ± 3.716
MCPO-rigid	2.941 ± 2.939
MCPO-deform	**1.798 ± 1.301**

mitted MCPO-deform as the Docker for the testing phase of the ReMIND2Reg sub-challenge.

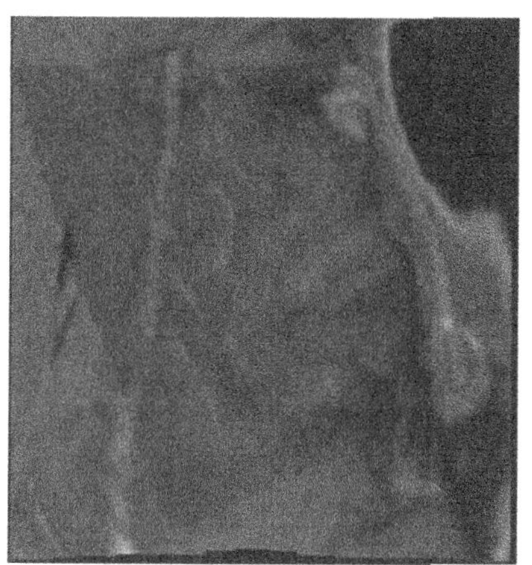

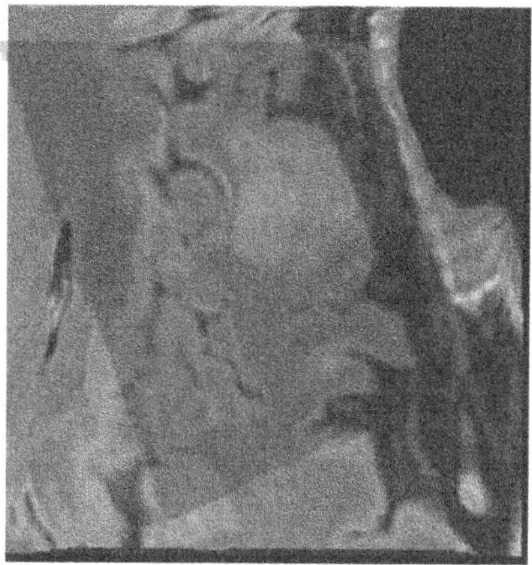

Fig. 4. Visualization result of MRI-US fusion for the large deformation case before (left) and after (right) registration using MCPO-deform.

Team	Rank		$ceT_1 \rightarrow$ iUS		$T_2 \rightarrow$ iUS	
	#	Score	TRE(%) ↓	TRE30(%)↓	TRE(%)↓	TRE30 (%) ↓
next-gen-nn	**1**	**0.911 (0.017)**	**2.9 (1.4)**	**2.0**	3.2 (1.9)	**2.2**
honkamj	2	0.905 (0.027)	3.2 (1.1)	2.5	**2.9 (1.0)**	2.3
VROC	3	0.566 (0.048)	3.9 (2.1)	2.8	3.3 (1.5)	2.7
lichlo	4	0.538 (0.039)	3.8 (1.3)	2.9	3.4 (1.2)	2.9
Initialization	5	0.199 (0.027)	5.1 (1.6)	4.0	5.1 (1.6)	4.0
noboby	6	0.181 (0.027)	5.2 (1.7)	4.0	5.2 (1.8)	4.1

Fig. 5. Results of methods in the test phase of ReMIND2Reg Sub-challenge. Reported by the organizer.

Test Phase of ReMIND2Reg Sub-challenge. Upon submission the Docker to the test phase, the organizer uniformly tested all participating teams' results, as illustrated in the figure. The competition officially introduced an additional metric, TRE30, defined as the 30th percentile of the TRE values computed across all landmarks, which further quantifies the registration performance after excluding potential outlier cases.

As shown in the Fig. 5[1], the MCPO-deform, corresponding to the results of team Next-gen-nn, achieves superior performance across most evaluation metrics. It should also be noted that the method from the second-placed team also demonstrates highly competitive registration accuracy. After normalizing all results, the proposed method attained a final score of 0.911 (out of 1.0), securing first place in the ReMIND2Reg Sub-challenge by a narrow margin. This outcome further validates that the proposed method exhibits enhanced generalization capability for preoperative-to-intraoperative registration and can effectively adapt to diverse and complex clinical scenarios.

4 Conclusion

The application of the proposed MCPO method to the Learn2Reg 2025 challenge shows that a multilevel optimization strategy using only a small amount of learning can quickly and accurately achieve the registration between multimodal medical images with large deformations. Meanwhile, the method proposed in this paper achieves promising results in Resect dataset, which illustrates the generality of the method for multimodal medical image registration.

Acknowledgments. Thanks all the organizers of the MICCAI 2025 Learn2Reg challenge. This work was supported by the National Natural Science Foundation of China under Grant U22B2050, 62425305, and 62221002.

References

1. Dorent, R., et al.: The Brain Resection Multimodal Image Registration (ReMIND2Reg) 2025 Challenge. arXiv preprint arXiv:2508.09649 (2025)
2. Balakrishnan, G., Zhao, A., Sabuncu, M. R., et al.: An unsupervised learning model for deformable medical image registration. In: 2018 IEEE/CVF Conference on Computer Vision and Pattern Recognition, Salt Lake City, UT, USA, pp. 9252–9260 (2018)
3. Zhang, H., Chen, X., Hu, R., et al.: MemWarp: discontinuity-preserving cardiac registration with memorized anatomical filters. In: Medical Image Computing and Computer Assisted Intervention–MICCAI 2024, pp. 671–681 (2024)
4. Chen, X., et al.: Spatially covariant image registration with text prompts. IEEE Trans. Neural Netw. Learn. Syst. **36**(7), 12925–12936 (2025)
5. Zhang, H., et al.: VoxelOpt: voxel-adaptive message passing for discrete optimization in deformable abdominal CT registration. In: Medical Image Computing and Computer Assisted Intervention–MICCAI 2025, pp. 672–683 (2025)
6. Chen, X., Diaz-Pinto, A., Ravikumar, N., Frangi, A.F.: Deep learning in medical image registration. Prog. Biomed. Eng. **3**(1), 012003 (2021)
7. Chen, X., Xia, Y., Ravikumar, N., Frangi, A.F.: A deep discontinuity-preserving image registration network. In: de Bruijne, M., et al. (eds.) MICCAI 2021. LNCS, vol. 12904, pp. 46–55. Springer, Cham (2021). https://doi.org/10.1007/978-3-030-87202-1_5

[1] https://learn2reg.grand-challenge.org/.

8. Siebert, H., Hansen, L., Heinrich, M.P.: Fast 3D registration with accurate optimisation and little learning for Learn2Reg 2021. In: Aubreville, M., Zimmerer, D., Heinrich, M. (eds.) Biomedical Image Registration, Domain Generalisation and Out-of-Distribution Analysis, MICCAI 2021. LNCS, vol. 13166. Springer, Cham (2022)
9. Heinrich, M., Jenkinson, M.: MIND: modality independent neighbourhood descriptor for multi-modal deformable registration. Med. Image Anal. **16**(7), 1423–1435 (2012)
10. Siebert, H., et al.: ConvexAdam: self-configuring dual-optimization-based 3D multitask medical image registration. IEEE Trans. Med. Imaging **44**(2), 738–748 (2024)
11. NiftyReg. https://github.com/KCL-BMEIS/niftyreg
12. Heinrich, M.P., Papież, B.W., Schnabel, J.A., Handels, H.: Non-parametric discrete registration with convex optimisation. In: Ourselin, S., Modat, M. (eds.) WBIR 2014. LNCS, vol. 8545, pp. 51–61. Springer, Cham (2014). https://doi.org/10.1007/978-3-319-08554-8_6
13. Juvekar, P., Dorent, R., Kögl, F., et al.: ReMIND: the brain resection multimodal imaging database. Nat. Sci. Data **11**, 494 (2024)
14. Daniel K., Matouš E., Marie-Charlotte D., et al.: CLEM-Reg: an automated point cloud based registration algorithm for correlative light and volume electron microscopy. bioRxiv 2023.05.11.540445 (2023)
15. Xiao, Y., Fortin, M., Unsgård, G., et al.: RE troSpective Evaluation of Cerebral Tumors (RESECT): a clinical database of pre-operative MRI and intra-operative ultrasound in low-grade glioma surgeries. Med. Phys. **44**(7), 3875–3882 (2017)
16. Wang, J., et al.: Unsupervised multimodal 3D medical image registration with multilevel correlation balanced optimization. arXiv preprint arXiv:2409.05040 (2024)

In Gradients We Trust: NGF-Driven Registration for ReMIND 2025

Thilo Sentker(✉) and Frederic Madesta

Institute for Applied Medical Informatics,
University Medical Center Hamburg-Eppendorf, Hamburg, Germany
{t.sentker,f.madesta}@uke.de

Abstract. We present a robust MRI–iUS registration pipeline designed to compensate for brain shift during surgery, developed for the ReMIND 2025 challenge. Our approach cleans up the data with modality-specific filtering (Gaussian for MRI, total variation for iUS) and aligns the images using a two-stage process: a coarse rigid alignment followed by an affine refinement. We rely on the Normalized Gradient Fields (NGF) loss to handle the difficult intensity differences between MRI and ultrasound, masking the optimization to focus strictly on relevant brain tissue. On the final test set, our method secured the 3rd rank, reducing the mean target registration error to 3.9 mm for T1 scans and 3.3 mm for T2 scans. This performance highlights the method's ability to recover alignment even without complex non-linear deformation models.

Keywords: ReMIND 2025 · MRI · iUS · Image Registration

1 Introduction

Surgical resection is a critical first step in the treatment of most brain tumors, with the extent of resection being the most important modifiable predictor of patient outcome. Neuronavigation systems have significantly improved intraoperative guidance by enabling surgeons to visualize the location of their instruments relative to the tumor and surrounding critical brain structures, as depicted in preoperative MRI. However, the accuracy of neuronavigation degrades over the course of surgery due to brain shift, a combination of intraoperative brain deformation and tissue resection, which results in spatial misalignment between preoperative images and the current intraoperative anatomy. Consequently, surgeons may be left without precise image guidance during the later stages of resection.

To address this challenge, intraoperative 3D ultrasound (iUS) provides a fast, radiation-free imaging modality capable of capturing the current state of the brain in real time. Registering iUS with preoperative MRI enables updating of neuronavigation to compensate for brain shift and restore surgical accuracy. Within the context of the ReMIND 2025 challenge [1], we propose a robust multi-stage MRI–iUS registration pipeline based on our VROC framework. Our

J. Chen et al. (Eds.): Learn2Reg 2025, LNCS 16254, pp. 12–16, 2026.
https://doi.org/10.1007/978-3-032-25169-5_2

approach integrates modality-specific preprocessing with multi-resolution rigid pre-registration, followed by affine refinement, and employs a central mask-based optimization to enhance alignment in clinically relevant regions.

2 Methods

2.1 Data

We used only the validation set of ReMIND 2025, as the training set does not provide ground-truth annotations (e.g., landmarks) required for quantitative evaluation of registration performance. Consequently, hyperparameter optimization was performed exclusively via submissions to the validation leaderboard. The dataset consists of paired preoperative magnetic resonance imaging (T1- and T2-weighted MRI) volumes and intraoperative 3D ultrasound (iUS) volumes acquired during brain tumor resections, as described in [3]. No external data were used. Throughout our framework, iUS volumes served as the fixed images, while MRI volumes were treated as the moving images.

2.2 Preprocessing

Before registration, MRI and iUS volumes underwent modality-specific preprocessing to improve image quality and enhance inter-modality similarity. MRI volumes were smoothed with a Gaussian filter to suppress high-frequency noise while preserving anatomical boundaries, whereas iUS volumes were denoised using total variation filtering to mitigate speckle artifacts without blurring edges. Finally, all images were standardized using z-score normalization.

2.3 Mask Generation

To focus registration on anatomically relevant regions and reduce the impact of ultrasound artifacts, the pipeline employs an automatic mask generation procedure. This removes the need for manual intervention while excluding low-quality areas.

The fixed image mask is obtained by extracting the largest connected tissue component and applying binary erosion to reduce boundary artifacts. Very low-intensity regions are then excluded using a 5th percentile threshold, followed by morphological smoothing to refine mask boundaries.

Probe position is estimated from the distribution of low-intensity background voxels along image borders. By counting such voxels in the first and last slices of each axis, the acquisition direction is inferred. Based on this, regions nearest to the probe, where the iUS signal is often unstable, are excluded, while border continuity is preserved to avoid edge artifacts.

The final mask combines the tissue- and probe-based components, concentrating registration on high-quality tissue regions and suppressing artifacts such as acoustic shadows, reverberations, and acquisition padding. This approach is robust across different probe orientations and acquisition protocols, reducing the need for manual mask definition.

2.4 Registration Pipeline

Our registration framework is built on the VROC tool and operates in two sequential stages. The pipeline is optimized to handle both available MRI modalities (T1 and T2) and is schematically illustrated in Fig. 1.

In the first stage, rigid pre-registration is applied to correct large-scale pose differences between the preoperative MRI and the iUS volumes. This step employs a rigid transformation model with six degrees of freedom, accounting for translations and rotations. Alignment is driven by the normalized gradient fields (NGF) loss ([2], cf. Eq. (1)) and optimized in a multi-resolution scheme across four levels, corresponding to relative resolutions of 0.25, 0.5, 0.75, and 1.0, where NGF is defined as

$$\mathcal{L}_{\text{NGF}} = \frac{\sum_{i,j,k} \left(1 - \left(\nabla \hat{F}_{i,j,k} \cdot \nabla \hat{M}_{i,j,k}\right)^2\right) m_{i,j,k}}{\sum_{i,j,k} m_{i,j,k} + \epsilon} \tag{1}$$

with $\nabla \hat{F}_{i,j,k} = \frac{\nabla F_{i,j,k}}{|\nabla F_{i,j,k}|+\epsilon}$ and $\nabla \hat{M}_{i,j,k} = \frac{\nabla M_{i,j,k}}{|\nabla M_{i,j,k}|+\epsilon}$ are normalized gradient vectors of fixed and moving images at voxel (i, j, k). The gradients ∇F and ∇M are computed by forward differences,

$$|\nabla F| = \sqrt{(\partial_x F)^2 + (\partial_y F)^2 + (\partial_z F)^2 + \epsilon}, \tag{2}$$

and analogously for M. The dot product quantifies gradient alignment, m is the binary mask, and ϵ ensures numerical stability. If the initial NGF similarity between moving and fixed images is already below a threshold of 0.65, only three levels are used. Each level is optimized for 50 iterations.

In the second stage, affine registration refines the alignment to capture local effects such as scaling and shearing that may occur due to brain deformation. This stage employs a full 12-degree-of-freedom affine transformation, optimized using the NGF loss at a single, full-resolution level with 150 iterations. Together, these two stages enable robust hierarchical alignment of MRI and iUS volumes, addressing both coarse misalignment and more subtle intraoperative deformations.

2.5 Implementation Details

The pipeline was implemented using the VROC registration framework (Python & C++). Optimization employed a gradient-based method with a mask-constrained NGF loss. The registration framework provides flexible configuration options for affine transformation optimization, allowing selective control over individual degrees of freedom including translation, scaling, rotation, and shearing components. Each transformation parameter can be independently enabled or disabled, enabling constraint-specific registration scenarios where certain motion types are restricted or prohibited. The optimization process employs adaptive learning rate scheduling with support for both exponential decay and

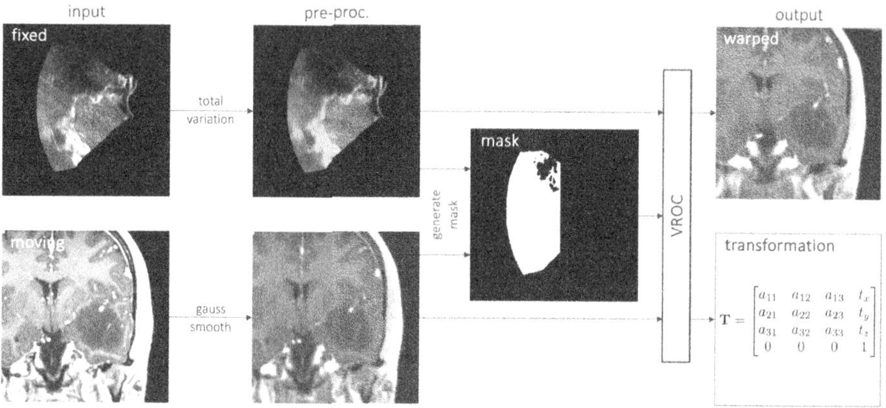

Fig. 1. Registration pipeline of our proposed approach.

plateau-based reduction strategies. An automatic step size adaptation mechanism monitors convergence behavior and dynamically reduces learning rates when optimization instability is detected. The framework implements configurable retry thresholds and minimum step size bounds to ensure robust convergence across diverse registration scenarios while maintaining computational efficiency through selective parameter optimization. All experiments were performed on an NVIDIA RTX A6000 GPU.

3 Results

During our internal development on the validation set, our best-performing configuration achieved a mean Target Registration Error (TRE) of 1.65 ± 0.47 mm. However, we observed that this setting was sensitive to small parameter changes. To ensure stability on unseen data, we deliberately selected a more robust configuration for the final submission, even though it yielded a slightly higher validation TRE of 2.00 ± 0.50 mm.

We submitted this configuration to the challenge organizers, who evaluated it on the held-out test set. Our method secured the 3rd rank overall, demonstrating the ability to correct the initial misalignment across both MRI modalities. For T1 scans, the mean TRE was reduced from a baseline of 5.1 mm down to 3.9 mm ($\pm$ 2.1 mm). We observed even better performance on T2-weighted scans, where the error dropped to 3.3 mm ($\pm$ 1.5 mm).

4 Discussion

Our results on the test set demonstrate a solid capability to handle brain shift, even without complex non-linear deformation models. The affine approach managed to capture enough of the global transformation to secure a top-3 ranking.

The fact that T2 scans registered better than T1 scans (3.3 mm vs 3.9 mm) suggests that the T2 contrast might naturally align better with the features visible in ultrasound, or perhaps the T1 contrast enhancement introduced gradients that confused the optimizer slightly.

We also noticed a distinct generalization gap. While our internal validation tests showed errors around 2 mm, the test set errors rose to roughly 3.3–3.9 mm. This jump is a reminder that real-world clinical data is unpredictable; the test cases likely included larger initial displacements or more complex deformations than the validation subset. However, because we prioritized a stable configuration during development, our method avoided catastrophic failures on these harder cases; it just yielded slightly higher errors, which is a necessary trade-off for clinical reliability.

Going forward, the obvious next step is to tackle the non-linear deformations. The affine transform handles the global shift, but it can't model the complex, localized warping that happens near the resection cavity. Adding a deformable stage to this pipeline would be the key to closing the gap in accuracy.

References

1. Dorent, R., et al.: The Brain Resection Multimodal Image Registration (ReMIND2Reg) 2025 Challenge (2025)
2. Haber, E., Modersitzki, J.: Intensity gradient based registration and fusion of multi-modal images. In: Larsen, R., Nielsen, M., Sporring, J. (eds.) MICCAI 2006. LNCS, vol. 4191, pp. 726–733. Springer, Heidelberg (2006). https://doi.org/10.1007/11866763_89
3. Juvekar, P., et al.: ReMIND: the brain resection multimodal imaging database. Sci. Data **11**(1) (2024)

Gabor-Based Neighborhood Descriptor for MRI–iUS Brain Image Registration

Chen-Yun Huang[1](✉) and Chiou-Shann Fuh[2]

[1] School of Professional Education and Continuing Studies, National Taiwan University, Taipei, Taiwan
[2] Department of Computer Science and Information Engineering, National Taiwan University, Taipei, Taiwan
fuh@csie.ntu.edu.tw

Abstract. In neurosurgical procedures, brain shift following resection significantly reduces the accuracy of neuronavigation based on preoperative MRI. To address this, the ReMIND2Reg challenge aims to develop robust registration methods between preoperative multi-modal MRI (ceT1 or T2) and intraoperative post-resection 3D ultrasound (iUS). We propose an unsupervised, feature-based registration pipeline that utilizes Gabor filters for structural descriptor extraction, computes Pearson-based similarity with neighborhood analysis, applies multi-stage masking to focus on informative regions, and fits an affine deformation model optimized via Covariance Matrix Adaptation Evolution Strategy (CMA-ES). Our method is tailored to be CPU-efficient and requires no learning from labeled data. Evaluations on the ReMIND2Reg validation dataset show that our approach consistently improves alignment compared to the baseline (NiftyReg) and zero-displacement methods, achieving lower Target Registration Error (TRE) across all cases.

Keywords: ReMIND2Reg · Multi-modal registration · Intraoperative Ultrasound Images · MRI · Gabor filter · Neighborhood Descriptor

1 Introduction

1.1 ReMIND2Reg Challenge [1,2]

Brain tumor resection is a key determinant of patient outcome, and intraoperative neuronavigation plays an essential role in guiding surgeons. However, its accuracy deteriorates during surgery due to brain shift caused by tissue deformation and resection. To compensate for this, the ReMIND2Reg challenge focuses on registering preoperative MRI with post-resection 3D intraoperative ultrasound (iUS) [1,2].

The task involves two settings: (i) iUS to contrast-enhanced T1-weighted MRI (ceT1), and (ii) iUS to T2-weighted MRI. Since not all MRI sequences are available for each patient, methods must flexibly handle either ceT1 or T2. The dataset includes 99 training patients (155 image pairs) and 5 validation patients (10 pairs), with private test cases used for final ranking.

J. Chen et al. (Eds.): Learn2Reg 2025, LNCS 16254, pp. 17–23, 2026.
https://doi.org/10.1007/978-3-032-25169-5_3

1.2 Related Work

The official baseline, NiftyReg [3], applies symmetric block matching with normalized cross-correlation (NCC) as the similarity measure, ensuring inverse consistency through Least Trimmed Squares updates.

Attribute-based methods such as DRAMMS [4,5] extract multi-scale, multi-orientation Gabor responses and weight correspondences via Mutual-Saliency to enhance robustness, combined with a diffeomorphic free-form deformation model optimized using Markov Random Fields.

More recent approaches, e.g., Multilevel Correlation Balanced Optimization (MCBO) [6,7], leverage the Modality Independent Neighborhood Descriptor with self-similarity context (MIND-SSC) [8] to construct displacement space volumes and optimize consistency across scales. These works highlight the importance of robust descriptors and multi-scale correlation modeling in cross-modality registration.

2 Methods

In this section, we describe our unsupervised registration pipeline, which consists of the following four stages: 1) extracting features with Gabor filters, 2) computing Pearson similarity to neighbors 3) masking non-informative regions, 4) pair-wise matching with affine model, and 5) optimizing results with Covariance Matrix Adaptation Evolution Strategy (CMA-ES).

2.1 Problem Setting

Let $I_{US}, I_{MR} : \Omega \subset \mathbb{Z}^3 \to \mathbb{R}$ denote the fixed iUS and the moving MR image, defined on the voxel lattice Ω. We estimate an affine transform

$$T_\theta(x) = Ax + b, \quad A \in \mathbb{R}^{3\times3},\ b \in \mathbb{R}^3, \tag{1}$$

and evaluate similarity only within a mask $M : \Omega \to \{0, 1\}$ (binary, but can be relaxed to $[0, 1]$).

2.2 Neighbor Set (MIND-Style)

We adopt a von Neumann metric shell of radius r as in MIND:

$$\mathcal{N}_r = \{\, \Delta \in \mathbb{Z}^3 \mid \|\Delta\|_1 = r \,\}. \tag{2}$$

In our implementation $r = 3$, yielding $|\mathcal{N}_3| = 38$ offset channels (of types $(3, 0, 0)$: 6, $(2, 1, 0)$: 24, $(1, 1, 1)$: 8; permutations and sign-flips included).

2.3 Per-frequency, Orientation-Channel Descriptor

For each spatial frequency $f \in \{1, \ldots, F\}$ and orientation $\phi \in \{1, \ldots, R\}$, let $\psi_{f,\phi}$ be a 3D Gabor kernel and

$$r_{f,\phi}(x) = (I * \psi_{f,\phi})(x). \tag{3}$$

Depending on the output mode, we form the orientation-channel vector $g^{(f)}(x) \in \mathbb{R}^R$ by

$$g_\phi^{(f)}(x) = \operatorname{Im} r_{f,\phi}(x) \tag{4}$$

so that the *orientation* dimension is preserved, while frequency is handled separately (next).

2.4 Offset-Wise Similarity per Frequency

For an offset $\Delta \in \mathcal{N}_r$, we compute a similarity between the orientation vectors at x and $x + \Delta$ *for each frequency*:

$$c_f(x, \Delta) = \frac{\langle g^{(f)}(x) - \bar{g}^{(f)}(x),\, g^{(f)}(x + \Delta) - \bar{g}^{(f)}(x + \Delta)\rangle}{\|g^{(f)}(x) - \bar{g}^{(f)}(x)\|\, \|g^{(f)}(x + \Delta) - \bar{g}^{(f)}(x + \Delta)\|}, \tag{5}$$

where $\bar{g}^{(f)}(x)$ is the mean over orientation channels.

Frequency Averaging After Similarity. As in our implementation, the offset-channel descriptor $m(x) \in \mathbb{R}^{|\mathcal{N}_r|}$ is obtained by *averaging the per-frequency similarities*:

$$m(x) = \frac{1}{F} \sum_{f=1}^{F} c_f(x, \Delta), \qquad \Delta \in \mathcal{N}_r. \tag{6}$$

This formulation emphasizes directional consistency across orientation channels and was found empirically to provide stable optimization. To stabilize local similarity, each offset channel is smoothed by a Gaussian filter

2.5 Mask

The mask M combines ultrasound background removal, Laplacian-variance gating, and a similarity-variance gate:

$$M(x) = M_{\text{US-zero}}(x)\, M_{\text{VarLap}}(x)\, M_{\text{VarSim}}(x). \tag{7}$$

The Laplacian variance threshold for iUS images was set to 0.2. The similarity variance threshold was set to 1.0 for iUS images and 0.01 for MR images. All thresholds were empirically determined on the training cases.

2.6 Registration Similarity and Objective

Given an affine T_θ in Eq. (1), we compare the fixed iUS descriptor and the warped MR descriptor *across offset channels* using Pearson correlation, followed by a monotone mapping $\varphi(\rho) = \exp(\rho) - 1$ (to stabilize optimization and accentuate high-correlation regions.):

$$s(x;\theta) = \varphi\left(\frac{\left\langle \tilde{m}^{US}(x) - \overline{\tilde{m}^{US}},\ \tilde{m}^{MR}(T_\theta(x)) - \overline{\tilde{m}^{MR}} \right\rangle}{\left\| \tilde{m}^{US}(x) - \overline{\tilde{m}^{US}} \right\| \left\| \tilde{m}^{MR}(T_\theta(x)) - \overline{\tilde{m}^{MR}} \right\|}\right), \tag{8}$$

where the bar denotes the mean over the offset-channel dimension. The masked objective we maximize is

$$\mathcal{S}(\theta) = \sum_{x \in \Omega} M(x)\, s(x;\theta). \tag{9}$$

2.7 Affine Parameterization and Warping

We adopt a two-stage optimization: first optimize a translation-dominant affine, then a Jacobian-normalized affine. The latter enforces an *incompressibility constraint* by normalizing $\det(A) = 1$, thus preserving tissue volume. This formulation retains shear and anisotropic distortion while discarding global hydrostatic scaling. Warping uses trilinear interpolation centered at the image center.

Optimization in both stages is performed using CMA-ES. In the first stage, the initial step size was set to 2.0, with a population size of 18 and 40 iterations. In the second stage, the initial step size was set to 1.0, with a population size of 6 and 80 iterations. For the second stage, parameter-wise standard deviations were used to constrain scaling, rotation, and shear components, improving stability during fine refinement.

Parameter-wise standard deviations were defined such that a unit perturbation would induce approximately a one-voxel displacement at the image boundary. This normalization ensures a comparable scale across translation, rotation, shear, and scaling parameters, promoting stable optimization.

2.8 Computing Infrastructure

Submissions were evaluated in the organizers' environment: Ubuntu 24.04 with an AMD EPYC-Milan CPU (16 cores @ 2 GHz), 60 GB RAM, and NVIDIA A100 GPU (20 GB), using CUDA 12.2, driver 535.247.01, and Docker 27.5.1. Local development and validation were performed on a Windows 11 workstation with an Intel Core i5-1230U CPU and 16 GB RAM.

3 Results

To evaluate quantitative performance, we submitted the estimated deformation fields to the ReMIND2Reg validation server, which returns the Target Registration Error (TRE) in millimeters. The spatial resolution of the dataset is 0.5 mm per voxel. As a baseline, we also report the TRE provided by the organizers for NiftyReg and zero displacement (i.e., no registration). The detailed results for all validation cases are summarized in Table 1, allowing a direct comparison of our method against the baselines.

Table 1. Comparison with NiftyReg. TRE in mm ↓.

Pair (with iUS)	NiftyReg	Zero Disp.	Ours
Case 98 ceT1	3.644	3.820	**1.528**
Case 98 T2	2.418	3.820	**1.385**
Case 99 ceT1	5.111	3.947	**2.060**
Case 99 T2	4.927	3.947	**2.928**
Case 100 ceT1	**1.838**	4.785	1.889
Case 100 T2	**1.885**	4.785	1.930
Case 101 ceT1	2.270	2.929	**1.380**
Case 101 T2	2.487	2.929	**2.437**
Case 102 ceT1	1.744	3.246	**1.261**
Case 102 T2	1.747	3.246	**1.662**
mean (ceT1)	2.921	3.745	**1.624**
std (ceT1)	1.288	0.639	**0.304**
mean (T2)	2.693	3.745	**2.068**
std (T2)	1.154	0.639	**0.552**
mean (overall)	2.807	3.745	**1.846**
std (overall)	1.228	0.639	**0.498**

4 Discussion

Our experiments show that the proposed Gabor–MIND descriptor, combined with mask-based gating and evolutionary optimization, can achieve consistent improvements over the NiftyReg baseline. The gain is especially evident in ceT1-to-iUS registration, suggesting that the orientation-channel similarity is more effective when contrast-enhanced anatomical structures are present. On T2, improvements are smaller but still positive, reflecting the modality's lower structural contrast.

The masking strategy played a crucial role in stabilizing optimization. By intersecting background erosion, Laplacian-variance filtering, and similarity-variance maps, we excluded unreliable regions (e.g., tumor cavities, bleeding, or far-field iUS artifacts) that otherwise caused local minima or unstable convergence. This heuristic shares the same spirit as Mutual Saliency, but avoids costly normalization and integrates seamlessly with the affine model.

Despite these strengths, our approach remains restricted to affine transformations and therefore cannot fully capture large, localized deformations. This limitation is particularly evident in post-resection cases with major tissue collapse. Moreover, the mask thresholds were tuned empirically and may not generalize optimally across all test cases.

Future extensions could combine our descriptor with a non-parametric deformation model such as free-form deformations, and explore hybrid optimizers that leverage both gradient information and evolutionary search. Although we adopted CMA-ES for robustness under non-differentiable settings (e.g., masking and SVD-based convolutions), a more systematic study of optimization strategies is still needed, and gradient-based methods may also be feasible with appropriate formulations. Another direction is adaptive masking or uncertainty weighting, so that reliable regions are emphasized without hand-crafted thresholds.

Finally, while we briefly tested MR–MR registration (T1 to T2) on a single case, the resulting affine alignment suggests that the descriptor is not limited to US–MR pairs. However, one case is insufficient for firm conclusions, and a more systematic evaluation is left for future work.

References

1. Juvekar, P., Dorent, R., Kögl, F., et al.: ReMIND: the brain resection multimodal imaging database. Sci. Data **11**(1), 494 (2024). https://doi.org/10.1038/s41597-024-03295-z
2. Dorent, R., et al.: The brain resection multimodal image registration (ReMIND2Reg) 2025 Challenge. arXiv preprint arXiv:2508.09649 (2025). https://doi.org/10.48550/arXiv.2508.09649
3. Drobny, D., Vercauteren, T., Ourselin, S., Modat, M.: Registration of MRI and iUS data to compensate brain shift using a symmetric block-matching based approach. In: Stoyanov, D., et al. (eds.) POCUS/BIVPCS/CuRIOUS/CPM 2018. LNCS, vol. 11042, pp. 172–178. Springer, Cham (2018). https://doi.org/10.1007/978-3-030-01045-4_21
4. Machado, I., et al.: Deformable MRI-ultrasound registration via attribute matching and mutual-saliency weighting for image-guided neurosurgery. In: Stoyanov, D., et al. (eds.) POCUS/BIVPCS/CuRIOUS/CPM -2018. LNCS, vol. 11042, pp. 165–171. Springer, Cham (2018). https://doi.org/10.1007/978-3-030-01045-4_20
5. Ou, Y., Sotiras, A., Paragios, N., Davatzikos, C.: DRAMMS: deformable registration via attribute matching and mutual-saliency weighting. Med. Image Anal. **15**(4), 622–639 (2011)
6. Wang, J., Chen, X., Zhang, Y., Liu, M., Wang, Y., Zhang, H.: Unsupervised multimodal 3D medical image registration with multilevel correlation balanced optimization. arXiv preprint arXiv:2409.05040 (2024)
7. Siebert, H., Großbröhmer, C., Hansen, L., Heinrich, M.P.: ConvexAdam: self-configuring dual-optimisation-based 3D multitask medical image registration. IEEE Trans. Med. Imaging **44**(2), 738–748 (2025). https://doi.org/10.1109/TMI.2024.3462248
8. Heinrich, M.P., et al.: MIND: modality independent neighbourhood descriptor for multi-modal deformable registration. Med. Image Anal. **16**(7), 1423–1435 (2012)

9. Chen, J., et al.: Beyond the LUMIR challenge: the pathway to foundational registration models. arXiv preprint arXiv:2505.24160 (2025)
10. Xiao, Y., et al.: Evaluation of MRI to ultrasound registration methods for brain shift correction: the CuRIOUS2018 challenge. IEEE Trans. Med. Imaging **39**(3), 777–786 (2020)
11. Liu, Q., Leung, H.: Tensor-based descriptor for image registration via unsupervised network. In: Int. Conf. on Information Fusion (Fusion), pp. 1–7. IEEE, Xi'an (2017). https://doi.org/10.23919/ICIF.2017.8009689
12. Hansen, N., Ostermeier, A.: Completely derandomized self-adaptation in evolution strategies. Evol. Comput. **9**(2), 159–195 (2001)

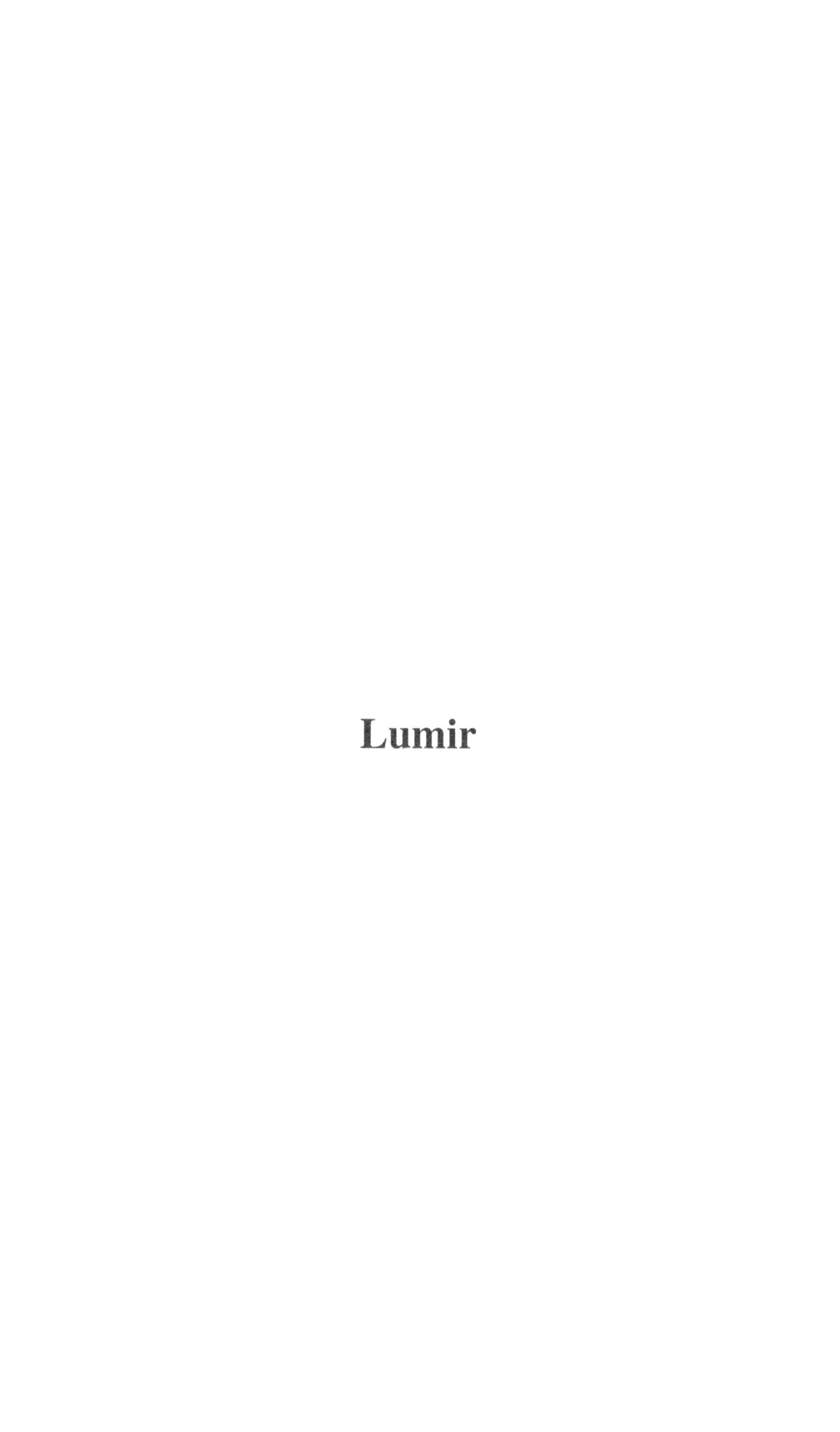

Lumir

Zero-Shot Multi-Contrast Brain MRI Registration by Intensity Randomizing T1-Weighted MRI (LUMIR25)

Hengjie Liu[1,2], Yimeng Dou[3], Di Xu[1], Xinyi Fu[1], Dan Ruan[2], and Ke Sheng[1](✉)

[1] University of California, San Francisco, San Francisco CA, USA
ke.sheng@ucsf.edu
[2] University of California, Los Angeles, Los Angeles CA, USA
[3] University of Wisconsin, Madison, Madison WI, USA

Abstract. In this paper, we present our submission to the LUMIR25 task of Learn2Reg 2025, which ranked 1st overall on the test set. Extended from LUMIR24, this year's task focuses on zero-shot registration under domain shifts (e.g., high-field MRI, pathological brains, and various MRI contrasts), while the training data comprises only in-domain T1-weighted brain MRI. We start with a meticulous analysis of LUMIR24 winners to identify the main contributors to strong monomodal registration performance. We highlight the importance of registration-specific inductive biases, including multi-resolution pyramids, inverse and group consistency, topological preservation or diffeomorphism, and correlation-based correspondence establishment. To further generalize to diverse contrasts, we employ three simple but effective strategies: (i) a multimodal loss based on the modality-independent neighborhood descriptor (MIND), (ii) intensity randomization for unseen contrast augmentation, and (iii) lightweight instance-specific optimization (ISO) on feature encoders at inference time. On the validation set, the proposed approach substantially improves T1–T2 registration accuracy, demonstrating robust cross-contrast generalization without relying on explicit image synthesis. These results suggest a practical step toward a registration foundation model that can leverage a single training domain yet remain robust across domain shifts.

Keywords: Deformable Image Registration · Multimodal Registration · Deep Learning · Domain Shift · Foundation Model · MIND

1 Introduction

The LUMIR24 challenge introduced a large-scale dataset for monomodal T1-weighted brain MRI registration [1, 2] and yielded fruitful results demonstrating the strength of deep learning in deformable image registration [3]. The winning method, SITReg [4], succeeded by emphasizing registration-specific inductive biases, including multi-resolution pyramids, by-construction inverse consistency (IC), group consistency (GC) and topological preservation, without resorting to complicated network architectures or

J. Chen et al. (Eds.): Learn2Reg 2025, LNCS 16254, pp. 27–36, 2026.
https://doi.org/10.1007/978-3-032-25169-5_4

advanced computation blocks such as Transformers or Mamba. The best-performing baseline, vector field attention (VFA) [5], was also notable for using a deterministic module to extract displacement directly from correlation features. Their success resonates with the recent studies that argue registration-specific designs matter more than choices of computation blocks [6–9]. Building on these insights, we closely examined the LUMIR24 leaders to identify the key "recipe" for strong monomodal registration.

As LUMIR25 shifts toward a foundation model capable of zero-shot registration while being trained only on T1-weighted images, we adopt three simple yet effective strategies to handle multimodal settings: (i) a multimodal loss based on the modality-independent neighborhood descriptor (MIND) [10]; (ii) intensity augmentation using smooth randomized mappings, and (iii) lightweight instance-specific optimization (ISO) applied only to the feature encoders with deformation prediction modules frozen.

2 Methods

2.1 Key Components for Monomodal Registration (LUMIR24)

We start by investigating key registration-specific design choices that are critical to registration performance inspired by [4–7, 11]. These include the multiresolution pyramid, correlation calculation, and inverse consistency. We design a unified framework to test the contribution of each component, as detailed in Fig. 1 and Table 1. Additional implementation details can be found in [8] and in our code repository: https://github.com/HengjieLiu/Unsupervised-DL-DIR-Revisited.

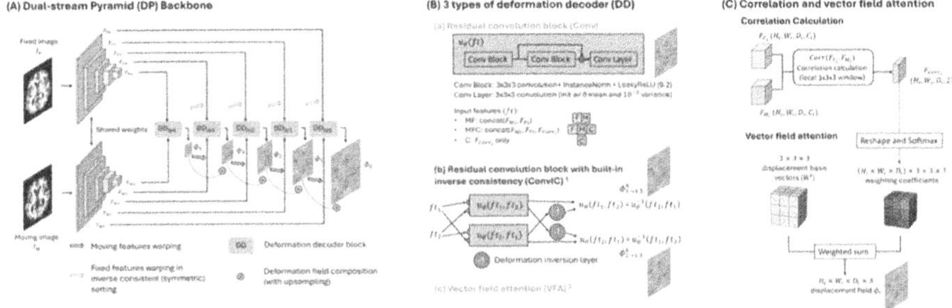

Fig. 1. (A) The standardized dual-stream pyramid (DP) backbone for registration. (B) Three types of deformation decoders. (C) Illustration of correlation calculation and vector field attention.

The registration results on LUMIR24 validation set are shown in Table 2. The multiresolution pyramid is key to achieving significantly better accuracy compared with VoxelMorph [12] and TransMorph [13] baselines. The inverse-consistent (IC) variants further improve regularity, as indicated by a lower non-diffeomorphic volume (NDV) [14]. Further, the correlation-only variants, despite having fewer parameters, surpass their counterparts, highlighting the role of correlation in deformation estimation.

However, in practice, correlation layers are memory intensive. Under our GPU constraint (48 GB VRAM), scaling up a backbone without correlation outperformed a smaller correlation-based model. In addition, the group consistency (GC) loss and the NDV loss—introduced by last year's winner—were highly effective at reducing HD95 and NDV, respectively, as shown in Table 3. Consequently, we still base our final model on the original SITReg without using correlation (similar to (b) DP-ConvIC-MF), and incorporates GC and NDV losses.

Table 1. High level summary of proposed methods and comparing methods.

Methods	Coarse -to-fine	Inverse consistency	Input features	Params (M) (encoder/decoder)
VoxelMorph	✗	✗	F M	0.3
TransMorph	✗	✗	F M	46.56
VFA	✓	✗	C	2.01
SITReg	✓	✓	F M	15.08
(a) DP-Conv-MF	✓	✗	F M	(0.51/2.35) 2.85
(a) DP-Conv-MFC	✓	✗	F M C	(0.51/2.66) 3.17
(a) DP-Conv-C	✓	✗	C	(0.51/1.49) 1.99
(b) DP-ConvIC-MF	✓	✓	F M	(0.51/2.35) 2.85
(b) DP-ConvIC-C	✓	✓	C	(0.51/1.80) 2.31
(c) DP-VFA	✓	✗	C	(0.51/0.28) 0.79

Table 2. Results on LUMIR24 validation set.

Methods	Dice ↑	HD95 ↓	TRE ↓	NDV (%) ↓
VoxelMorph	0.7186 ± 0.0340	3.9821	3.1545	1.1836
TransMorph	0.7594 ± 0.0319	3.5074	2.4225	0.3509
(a) DP-Conv-MF	0.7713 ± 0.0290	3.3534	2.4676	0.4158
(a) DP-Conv-MFC	0.7730 ± 0.0291	3.3566	2.4449	0.4672
(a) DP-Conv-C	0.7747 ± 0.0295	3.3666	2.4135	0.3795
(b) DP-ConvIC-MF	0.7717 ± 0.0288	3.3489	2.3660	0.0310
(b) DP-ConvIC-C	0.7724 ± 0.0288	3.3873	2.3357	0.0309
(c) DP-VFA	0.7764 ± 0.0284	3.2157	2.4420	0.0540
VFA	0.7726 ± 0.0286	3.2127	2.4949	0.0788
SITReg	0.7742 ± 0.0291	3.3039	2.3112	0.0231
SITReg (GC/NDV)	**0.7805 ± 0.0287**	**3.1187**	**2.3005**	**0.0025**

2.2 Extension to Multimodal Registration (LUMIR25)

MIND Loss. Our first adaptation for multimodal registration is to use a MIND-based similarity loss [10] instead of normalized cross correlation (NCC). The loss function is

$$Loss = \lambda_1 L_{sim} + \lambda_2 L_{smooth} + \lambda_3 L_{GC} + \lambda_4 L_{NDV}, \tag{1}$$

where $\lambda_1 = 1$ for NCC and $\lambda_1 = 10$ for MIND, $\lambda_2 = 1$ with a diffusion regularizer, and $\lambda_3 = 40$ and $\lambda_4 = 1e - 5$ as in SITReg. Although all LUMIR24 participants used NCC loss [3], we find that MIND performs competitively with NCC on LUMIR24 (Table 3). Notably, it improves TRE, which is expected since MIND is sensitive to edge and corner structures. Adding GC and NDV losses further improves accuracy (Dice and HD95) for MIND as well.

Table 3. Comparison of NCC loss vs. MIND loss on LUMIR24 validation set.

Methods	Dice ↑	HD95 ↓	TRE ↓	NDV (%) ↓
SITReg-NCC	0.7735 ± 0.0285	3.3183	2.3266	0.0267
SITReg-NCC (GC/NDV)	**0.7798 ± 0.0289**	3.1296	2.3102	**0.0024**
SITReg-MIND	0.7705 ± 0.0276	3.3781	**2.2702**	0.1045
SITReg-MIND (GC/NDV)	0.7761 ± 0.0290	**3.0685**	2.3139	0.0067

Intensity Augmentation. Intensity augmentation has been widely used in domain generalization for medical image segmentation [15]. To mimic inter-sequence appearance shifts while preserving anatomical structures, we apply a smooth, randomized point-wise intensity remapping to each T1-weighted training volume. Specifically, we define a smooth intensity remapping function $g(x)$ using a shape-preserving piecewise-cubic Hermite interpolant (PCHIP), which yields a C^1 mapping. We parameterize g by n_{knots} control points $\{(x_i, y_i)\}_{i=1}^{n_{knots}}$ over the intensity range [0, 255], where the knot locations x_i are uniformly spaced. We fix the endpoints to satisfy $g(0) = 0$ and $g(255) = 255$, and randomly sample the remaining $n_{knots} - 2$ interior values y_i. We then discretize g at integer intensities to obtain a 256-entry lookup table $T : \{0, \ldots, 255\} \rightarrow \{0, \ldots, 255\}$, and apply it voxelwise via $v' = T(v)$. To avoid degenerate contrast collapse, we reject candidates whose post-mapping histograms show saturated bins with a preset threshold. We empirically set $n_{knots} = 6$, but further optimization could yield additional gains. Examples of augmented images are shown in Fig. 2. The augmented images can resemble other contrasts such as T2-weighted images. In total, we precomputed 2,000 mappings and applied them randomly during training.

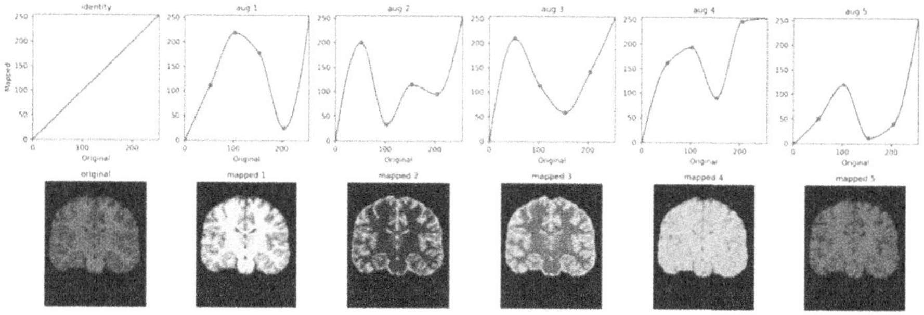

Fig. 2. Intensity randomization examples for multimodal emulation. Aug #4 will be rejected.

ISO Strategy. In LUMIR24, SITReg outperformed other methods on in-domain T1–T1 registration without relying on instance-specific optimization (ISO). However, ISO has been reported to enhance robustness for zero-shot tasks [3, 16]. While ISO can further decrease the pairwise registration loss at inference time, it may overfit to intensity matching (i.e., the similarity loss). Empirically, we observed better Dice and HD95 with strong GC regularization, whereas pairwise ISO can break away from this regularization and slightly worsen Dice and HD95. Therefore, we did not use ISO for T1–T1 tasks and experimented with ISO for other modalities. To mitigate overfitting, we apply ISO only to the feature encoder (ISO-fe) while keeping the deformation decoder frozen. This is reasonable because the decoder has already been exposed to diverse feature styles through augmentation, whereas adapting the encoder can better accommodate unseen intensity profiles while limiting the risk of overfitting. Moreover, ISO-fe updates only 22% of the total parameters compared with ISO-full. We ran both ISO-fe and ISO-full for 20 steps using the loss function in Eq. 1, while omitting the GC term.

2.3 Submitted Method

Our final submission integrates two models to maximize performance under the challenge evaluation metrics. For T1–T1 registration, we use SITReg-NCC (GC/NDV) without ISO, as it performs slightly better than SITReg-MIND (GC/NDV). For all other imaging contrast pairs, we use SITReg-MIND-Aug (GC/NDV), with ISO-fe applied at inference time.

The models were implemented in PyTorch 2.5.1, and all training was conducted on NVIDIA RTX 6000 Ada GPUs with 48 GB of memory. Group consistency training required three GPUs to process three image pairs in parallel, whereas ISO was performed on a single GPU.

3 Results

The validation set comprises 36 registration pairs in total:

- 18 in-domain (ID) T1–T1 pairs (9 evaluated with contour-based metrics and 9 with landmark-based metrics),
- 9 out-of-domain (OD) high-field T1–T1 pairs (evaluated with contour-based metrics),
- 9 multimodal (MM) T1–T2 pairs (evaluated with contour-based metrics).

3.1 Ablation on Proposed Strategies

Table 4 reports the validation results on the three subsets (ID, OD, and MM), presenting an ablation study that highlights the contribution of each component. The key findings are as follows.

Table 4. Registration results on the validation set across three subsets, illustrating the effects of the proposed components: MIND similarity, intensity augmentation (Aug), and instance-specific optimization (ISO). All SITReg variants are trained with GC and NDV losses.

(a) In-domain T1 - T1 (9 contour-based+9 landmark-based=18 pairs)

Methods	Dice ↑	HD95 ↓	TRE ↓	NDV (%) ↓
SynthMorph (Baseline)	0.7262 ± 0.0133	3.5763 ± 0.1963	2.6099 ± 0.3627	0.0000 ± 0.0000
SITReg-NCC	**0.7816 ± 0.0171**	3.1091 ± 0.2445	2.3103 ± 0.2705	0.0023 ± 0.0005
SITReg-MIND	0.7796 ± 0.0170	3.1102 ± 0.2363	2.3358 ± 0.3165	0.0075 ± 0.0008
SITReg-MIND-Aug	0.7791 ± 0.0159	**3.0974 ± 0.2339**	2.2988 ± 0.2993	0.0069 ± 0.0009
SITReg-MIND-Aug + ISO-full	0.7722 ± 0.0156	3.3213 ± 0.2695	**2.2615 ± 0.3068**	0.0047 ± 0.0006
SITReg-MIND-Aug + ISO-fe	0.7730 ± 0.0152	3.2721 ± 0.2488	2.2948 ± 0.3024	0.0059 ± 0.0009

(b) Out-of-domain (high-field) T1–T1 (9 pairs)

Methods	Dice ↑	HD95 ↓	NDV (%) ↓
SynthMorph (Baseline)	0.6888 ± 0.0202	3.9061 ± 0.4199	0.0000 ± 0.0000
SITReg-NCC	**0.7652 ± 0.0157**	3.1738 ± 0.3244	0.0027 ± 0.0001
SITReg-MIND	0.7610 ± 0.0148	**3.1648 ± 0.3097**	0.0079 ± 0.0008
SITReg-MIND-Aug	0.7595 ± 0.0145	3.2032 ± 0.2845	0.0077 ± 0.0006
SITReg-MIND-Aug + ISO-full	0.7575 ± 0.0119	3.3525 ± 0.2937	0.0069 ± 0.0008
SITReg-MIND-Aug + ISO-fe	0.7560 ± 0.0134	3.3192 ± 0.3296	0.0065 ± 0.0009

(c) Multimodal T1 - T2 (9 pairs)

Methods	Dice ↑	HD95 ↓	NDV (%) ↓
SynthMorph (Baseline)	0.6888 ± 0.0244	3.2489 ± 0.3091	0.0000 ± 0.0000
SITReg-NCC	0.3564 ± 0.0192	6.0990 ± 0.3403	0.0007 ± 0.0003
SITReg-MIND	0.3691 ± 0.0175	5.9121 ± 0.4434	0.0097 ± 0.0021
SITReg-MIND-Aug	0.7165 ± 0.0238	**2.7409 ± 0.1777**	0.0044 ± 0.0008
SITReg-MIND-Aug + ISO-full	0.7236 ± 0.0276	2.8723 ± 0.1907	0.0049 ± 0.0007
SITReg-MIND-Aug + ISO-fe	**0.7241 ± 0.0284**	2.8328 ± 0.1977	0.0048 ± 0.0007

MIND vs. NCC. NCC remains competitive for monomodal T1–T1 registration. For both in-domain and out-of-domain T1–T1, SITReg-NCC achieves the best Dice, while differences in HD95 and TRE vary across methods and require further validation on larger test sets. Using MIND loss with ISO can improve landmark-related alignment (TRE), indicating better point-wise correspondence; however, this does not translate into higher Dice, suggesting a potential trade-off between landmark fidelity and volumetric overlap.

Intensity Augmentation. Intensity augmentation is essential for cross-contrast generalization. Without augmentation, both SITReg-NCC and SITReg-MIND perform poorly on multimodal T1–T2 registration. Introducing the proposed intensity randomization markedly improves robustness. SITReg-MIND-Aug shows strong T1–T2 performance and consistently outperforms the SynthMorph [17] baseline across all three validation subsets, highlighting the effectiveness of learning from real T1 anatomy while simulating diverse contrast appearances.

ISO for T1–T1. ISO is not beneficial for T1–T1. Applying ISO to monomodal T1–T1 tends to slightly degrade Dice and HD95 in both in-domain and out-of-domain settings, suggesting that pairwise ISO may overfit to the similarity objective and partially undermine the benefits induced by GC regularization.

ISO for T1–T2. Encoder-only ISO is the safer choice for multimodal registration. For T1–T2, both ISO-full and ISO-fe improve Dice over SITReg-MIND-Aug, but can increase HD95. Compared with ISO-full, ISO-fe provides a better trade-off, achieving larger Dice gains while degrading HD95 less. This supports adapting only the encoder to accommodate unseen intensity profiles while keeping the deformation decoder frozen.

3.2 Validation Results of the Final Submission

Our final validation results are shown in Table 5. For reference, we also report SynthSR-based baselines, which synthesize T1-like images from T2-weighted inputs [18] and then apply a monomodal registration model (SITReg or VFA). Our proposed method performs slightly worse than the SynthSR-based approaches on T1–T2 registration, but the gap is small.

Table 5. Registration results on the LUMIR25 validation set.

(a) Aggregated results.

Methods	Dice ↑	HD95 ↓	TRE ↓	NDV (%) ↓
Final submission	0.7570 ± 0.0322	3.0388 ± 0.2989	2.3099 ± 0.2704	0.0030 ± 0.0012
SITReg + synthSR	0.7610 ± 0.0281	2.9968 ± 0.3322	2.3102 ± 0.2707	0.0024 ±0.0004
VFA + synthSR	0.7536 ± 0.0260	3.1075 ± 0.3320	2.4956 ± 0.3783	0.0074 ±0.0050

(b) Subset results.

Methods	Dice(ID)	Dice(OD)	Dice(MM)	HD95(ID)	HD95(OD)	HD95(MM)
Final submission	0.7816	0.7652	0.7240	3.1095	3.1740	2.8329
SITReg + synthSR	0.7816	0.7652	0.7363	3.1096	3.1743	2.7065
VFA + synthSR	0.7744	0.7545	0.7320	3.2033	3.2963	2.8228

4 Discussion

The proposed method—SITReg backbone with GC/NDV regularization, MIND-based similarity, intensity randomization, and encoder-only ISO—enables multimodal registration despite being trained only on T1-weighted images. Overall, the recipe is simple, effective and robust. SITReg-MIND-Aug and both ISO variants consistently outperform SynthMorph, a strong contrast-invariant baseline that generalizes by training on synthetically generated label maps and images spanning diverse contrasts and shapes [17]. These gains could be attributed to the proposed real-image–anchored intensity randomization and/or to the strong registration-specific inductive biases (e.g., multi-resolution pyramids, inverse/group consistency) embedded in the SITReg framework. A more controlled ablation is needed to isolate the contribution of each factor. On the T1–T2 validation subset, the proposed method is slightly inferior to synthSR-based baselines. Still, it may be more robust when synthesis fails or hallucinates contrast, since our pipeline does not rely on an explicit synthesis model or a fixed intensity mapping. Overall, our study provides a practical step toward a "registration foundation model" for single-site (brain MRI) multi-modal registration, where a single training source can be leveraged to generalize to unseen domain shifts.

However, there remains a clear accuracy gap across in-domain, out-of-domain, and multimodal validation, indicating room for improvement. A better-designed augmentation scheme that includes local varying effects (e.g., bias fields, local contrast changes, and noise characteristics) and more realistic contrast mimicking may narrow this gap without introducing additional complexity of synthesis. In addition, correlation-based matching remains a promising direction for improving correspondence in challenging multimodal cases, but realizing its benefits at useful scales will require addressing memory constraints.

The final test results confirm that our submitted solution performs strongly for all T1–T1 registration tasks (both in-domain and out-of-domain), but falls short on multimodal tasks. The strong performance on T1–T1 tasks is attributed to the successful strategies in SITReg. Using MIND loss as we experimented or MIND features as in [19] can improve robustness to out-of-domain contrast variations, but may slightly reduce contour-matching metrics in this particular challenge. Nevertheless, these strategies may be beneficial for more diverse clinical scenarios. We also observe that MIND improves landmark matching (TRE) due to its structure-driven nature.

We further found that the effectiveness of ISO for bridging domain gaps, as reported in [16], needs further verification. In particular, ISO did not improve performance on the out-of-domain high-field validation subset, and we achieved strong out-of-domain T1–T1 results on diverse test sets without ISO. We suspect that pairwise ISO can overfit to intensity matching and partially undermine the benefits of regularization. Understanding when ISO becomes beneficial (i.e., how large a domain gap is needed and under what regularization scheme) remains an open question.

Finally, we want to highlight **the importance of registration-specific inductive biases**, including multi-resolution pyramids, inverse consistency, group consistency, topological preservation or diffeomorphism, and correlation-assisted correspondence establishment. *These ideas are not new, yet they are often overlooked or underexplored in many (if not most) trend-driven learning-based methods.* We also found the correlation-only models very promising. The idea was proposed fairly early in deep learning–based optical flow research [20]. Correlation-only variants can achieve strong results with fewer parameters than intensity-feature-only or hybrid models. Preliminary results (not included) further suggest that correlation-only models may require less training data and be less prone to overfitting to the similarity objective: in our experiments, intensity-feature–based models degrade considerably without regularization, whereas correlation-only models remain comparatively robust.

Acknowledgments. This study was funded by NIH (R01CA188300) and DOD (W81XWH2210044).

Disclosure of Interests. The authors have no competing interests to declare that are relevant to the content of this article.

References

1. Dufumier, B., Grigis, A., Victor, J., Ambroise, C., Frouin, V., Duchesnay, E.: OpenBHB: a large-scale multi-site brain MRI data-set for age prediction and Debiasing. NeuroImage. **263**, 119637 (2022). https://doi.org/10.1016/j.neuroimage.2022.119637
2. Taha, A., et al.: Magnetic resonance imaging datasets with anatomical fiducials for quality control and registration. Sci. Data. **10**, 449 (2023). https://doi.org/10.1038/s41597-023-02330-9
3. Chen, J., et al.: Beyond the LUMIR challenge: The pathway to foundational registration models, http: //arxiv.org/abs/2505.24160, (2025). https://doi.org/10.48550/arXiv.2505.24160.
4. Honkamaa, J., Marttinen, P.: SITReg: multi-resolution architecture for symmetric, inverse consistent, and topology preserving image registration. Mach. Learn. Biomed. Imaging. **2**, 2148–2194 (2024). https://doi.org/10.59275/j.melba.2024-276b
5. Liu, Y., Chen, J., Zuo, L., Carass, A., Prince, J.L.: Vector field attention for deformable image registration. J. Med. Imaging. **11**, 064001 (2024). https://doi.org/10.1117/1.JMI.11.6.064001
6. Heinrich, M.P.: Closing the gap between deep and conventional image registration using probabilistic dense displacement networks. In: Shen, D., et al. (eds.) Medical Image Computing and Computer Assisted Intervention–MICCAI 2019, pp. 50–58. Springer International Publishing, Cham (2019). https://doi.org/10.1007/978-3-030-32226-7_6
7. Jian, B., Pan, J., Ghahremani, M., Rueckert, D., Wachinger, C., Wiestler, B.: Mamba? Catch The Hype Or Rethink What Really Helps for Image Registration, http://arxiv.org/abs/2407.19274, (2024). https://doi.org/10.48550/arXiv.2407.19274.
8. Liu, H., Ruan, D., Sheng, K.: Unsupervised Deformable Image Registration Revisited: Enhancing Performance with Registration-Specific Designs. Presented at the Medical Imaging with Deep Learning - Short Papers April 12 (2025).
9. Jian, B., et al.: Disentangling Progress in Medical Image Registration: Beyond Trend-Driven Architectures towards Domain-Specific Strategies, http://arxiv.org/abs/2512.01913, (2025). https://doi.org/10.48550/arXiv.2512.01913.
10. Heinrich, M.P., et al.: MIND: modality independent neighbourhood descriptor for multi-modal deformable registration. Med. Image Anal. **16**, 1423–1435 (2012). https://doi.org/10.1016/j.media.2012.05.008
11. Kang, M., Hu, X., Huang, W., Scott, M.R., Reyes, M.: Dual-stream pyramid registration network. Med. Image Anal. **78**, 102379 (2022). https://doi.org/10.1016/j.media.2022.102379

12. Balakrishnan, G., Zhao, A., Sabuncu, M.R., Guttag, J., Dalca, A.V.: VoxelMorph: a learning framework for deformable medical image registration. IEEE Trans. Med. Imaging. **38**, 1788–1800 (2019). https://doi.org/10.1109/TMI.2019.2897538
13. Chen, J., Frey, E.C., He, Y., Segars, W.P., Li, Y., Du, Y.: TransMorph: transformer for unsupervised medical image registration. Med. Image Anal. **82**, 102615 (2022). https://doi.org/10.1016/j.media.2022.102615
14. Liu, Y., Chen, J., Wei, S., Carass, A., Prince, J.: On finite difference Jacobian computation in deformable image registration. Int. J. Comput. Vis. **132**, 3678–3688 (2024). https://doi.org/10.1007/s11263-024-02047-1
15. Su, Z., Yao, K., Yang, X., Huang, K., Wang, Q., Sun, J.: Rethinking data augmentation for single-source domain generalization in medical image segmentation. In: Proceedings of the Thirty-Seventh AAAI Conference on Artificial Intelligence and Thirty-Fifth Conference on Innovative Applications of Artificial Intelligence and Thirteenth Symposium on Educational Advances in Artificial Intelligence, pp. 2366–2374. AAAI Press (2023). https://doi.org/10.1609/aaai.v37i2.25332
16. Mok, T.C.W., et al.: Deformable medical image registration under distribution shifts with neural instance optimization. In: Cao, X., Xu, X., Rekik, I., Cui, Z., Ouyang, X. (eds.) Machine Learning in Medical Imaging, pp. 126–136. Springer Nature, Switzerland, Cham (2024). https://doi.org/10.1007/978-3-031-45673-2_13
17. Hoffmann, M., Billot, B., Greve, D.N., Iglesias, J.E., Fischl, B., Dalca, A.V.: Synth morph: learning contrast-invariant registration without acquired images. IEEE Trans. Med. Imaging. **41**, 543–558 (2022). https://doi.org/10.1109/TMI.2021.3116879
18. Iglesias, J.E., et al.: Joint super-resolution and synthesis of 1 mm isotropic MP-RAGE volumes from clinical MRI exams with scans of different orientation, resolution and contrast. NeuroImage. **237**, 118206 (2021). https://doi.org/10.1016/j.neuroimage.2021.118206
19. Honkamaa, J., Marttinen, P.: Strategies for Robust Deep Learning Based Deformable Registration, http://arxiv.org/abs/2510.23079, (2025). https://doi.org/10.48550/arXiv.2510.23079.
20. Dosovitskiy, A., et al.: FlowNet: learning optical flow with convolutional networks. In: In: 2015 IEEE International Conference on Computer Vision (ICCV), pp. 2758–2766. IEEE, Santiago (2015). https://doi.org/10.1109/ICCV.2015.316

Strategies for Robust Deep Learning Based Deformable Registration

Joel Honkamaa(✉) and Pekka Marttinen

Aalto University, Espoo, Finland
joel.honkamaa@aalto.fi

Abstract. Deep learning based deformable registration methods have become popular in recent years. However, their ability to generalize beyond training data distribution can be poor, significantly hindering their usability. LUMIR brain registration challenge for Learn2Reg 2025 aims to advance the field by evaluating the performance of the registration on contrasts and modalities different from those included in the training set. Here we describe our submission to the challenge, which proposes a very simple idea for significantly improving robustness by transforming the images into MIND feature space before feeding them into the model. In addition, a special ensembling strategy is proposed that shows a small but consistent improvement.

Keywords: Image registration · Deformable image registration · Multi-modal image registration · Deep learning · MIND

1 Introduction

Deep learning based medical image registration methods have emerged as a strong alternative for classical iterative methods, but their usability has been brought to question due to their potentially poor performance on data outside the training distribution [8]. However, the best methods submitted for the LUMIR MRI brain registration challenge organized as part of Learn2Reg 2024 showed strong robustness to domain shifts, failing only on out-of-distribution contrasts. LUMIR challenge for Learn2reg 2025 aims to advance the field particularly in this regard: For training, one is required to use the provided T1-weighted brain MRI images but the evaluation is performed on new contrasts or even modalities. This paper is an algorithm description of our submission to the challenge.

As our main contribution, we propose to transform the images using the MIND [5] transformation before feeding them into the model, while still using intra-modality similarity loss (normalized cross-correlation) as the training signal. While the MIND features contain less information than the original images, the transformation unifies the representation between different modalities, and the performance on in-domain images remains similar. Earlier MIND features or its variants have been used for evaluating multi-modal similarity (including in deep learning [1,4,6]) but to our knowledge they have not been used as an

J. Chen et al. (Eds.): Learn2Reg 2025, LNCS 16254, pp. 37–42, 2026.
https://doi.org/10.1007/978-3-032-25169-5_5

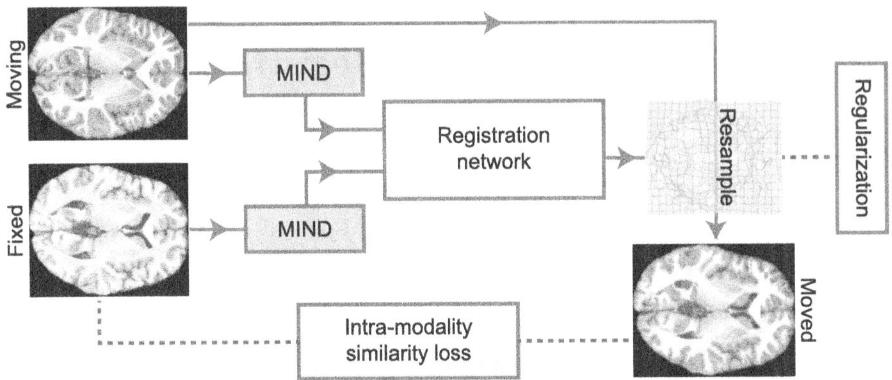

Fig. 1. Overview of the proposed main idea. The input images go through the MIND transformation before being fed to the registration network. As a result, the network learns to do multi-modal registration even though it is trained with an intra-modality similarity loss. The similarity loss is normalized cross-correlation. Also note that in practice the registration network predicts the deformation in both directions, and the losses are also computed for both directions.

input transformation in deep learning before. In addition, we propose a special ensembling strategy which still retains the diffeomorphic properties of the used backbone model (Fig. 1).

2 Background

MIND (Modality Independent Neighborhood Descriptor) [5] is a well-established and simple method for measuring multi-modal similarity. The method works by computing MIND features of both images and then taking some simple distance measure such as the mean absolute error or mean squared error between the resulting volumes. MIND encodes how similar a voxel's neighborhood is to its surrounding neighborhoods, not the absolute intensity values.

Given an offset r, the formula for computing a single MIND feature at location x can be written as

$$\mathrm{MIND}(x, r) = \exp\left(-\frac{D(I, x, x + r)}{V(I, x)}\right) \tag{1}$$

where $D(I, x, x + r)$ is the Gaussian-weighted sum of the squared differences between the patches around x and $x + r$

$$D(I, x, y) := \sum_{p \in P} \exp(-\frac{p^2}{\sigma^2})(I(x + p) - I(y + p))^2 \tag{2}$$

with P being large enough lattice around origin to incorporate most of the Gaussian, and $V(I, x)$ is local variance of I estimated as the mean of D in the six-neighborhood around x, giving $V(I, x) := \frac{1}{6} \sum_{n \in \mathcal{N}} D(I, x, x + n)$. Here, I refers to the image, and $\mathcal{N}$ is the six-neighborhood around origin. To compute MIND features, Eq. 1 is evaluated for each voxel and multiple offsets, and each voxel is associated with a feature vector consisting of those values. The six-neighborhood set is often used for the offsets as well, resulting in a six-dimensional feature vector.

3 Methods

3.1 Backbone

As a backbone architecture we use our work SITReg [7] which was used by the winning submission for Learn2Reg 2024. The architecture is by construction symmetric, inverse consistent, and produces diffeomorphic deformations. The overall architecture starts by extracting multiresolution features from both images independently using ResNet-style convolutional neural network. The architecture then recursively updates the deformation at each resolution starting from the lowest resolution. At each resolution stage, the features of that resolution are transformed by the deformation learned up to that point and are then used to predict a deformation update in symmetric manner. The update deformations are generated using constrained B-spline control points to ensure diffeomorphic predictions. See the paper for more details.

3.2 Input Transformation

The challenge requires the method to work on images of different contrast or modality from the training images. In general, the behavior of machine learning algorithms on inputs outside the training distribution is hard to predict, and for that reason we take the approach of trying to transform the images to some representation which contains less information than the original representation but is similar across contrasts and modalities. Preferably, mainly the structural information would be preserved. The MIND transformation described in Sect. 2 is a well-established and simple transformation that unifies different modalities. Note that unlike in the usual use case, we do not use the MIND transformation in computing the similarity loss which is instead computed with the original images using intra-modality loss. Since MIND features unify representation across modalities, the symmetric nature of the backbone architecture is still meaningful even for multi-modal registration. We use $\sigma = 0.5$ for the MIND transformation (Eq. 2) which performed the best in the original paper [5].

3.3 Ensembling

We train an ensemble of 5 models with different data generation seeds. For the final prediction we average the predicted update deformations at each registration stage of the SITReg multiresolution architecture. We perform averaging in the B-spline weight space to preserve the diffeomorphic properties of the architecture.

3.4 Further Details

We also use augmentations to help with generalization. We randomly apply Gaussian noise, Gaussian blur, sign inversion, and gamma correction to the input images.

We use normalized cross-correlation as a similarity metric. Due to the MIND input transformation, the network still learns to register images of different modality. For computing the similarity loss, we always use the original non-augmented images, and mask the background out. We regularize the predicted deformations with diffusion regularization (L^2 norm on displacements). While the original SITReg paper applied the losses only after the final stage of its multi-resolution architecture, we apply the loss also on intermediate stages to ensure consistent behavior across the trained model ensemble. However, we use very low loss weight of $\frac{1}{100}$ for the earlier stages.

While the SITReg backbone produces nearly perfectly diffeomorphic deformations, due to resampling errors tiny folding errors can still occur. To ensure a very high competency, we add non-diffeomorphic volume (NDV) [9] as an additional loss term for the final epochs. We also train with group consistency loss [3] for the final epochs. The loss encourages the composition of predicted deformations over image cycles to be identity mappings. Note that NDV and group consistency losses were also used in the winning submission of Learn2Reg 2024 which was also based on the SITReg architecture. The strategies are documented by the GitHub repository https://github.com/honkamj/SITReg.

The training setup is implemented in PyTorch and we trained the models with A100 and H100 GPUs using Adam as an optimizer. For the group consistency training included for final epochs we used 3 GPUs per training since the loss computation did not easily fit on a single GPU. The earlier epochs we trained on a single GPU.

4 Results

In Table 1 the results of the LUMIR 2025 validation set are shown for the different ablations. The dataset [2,10] used for training the network consists of T1-weighted brain MRI images. The validation set also consists of brain MRI images, but the out-of-domain set contains T1-weighted images from a different dataset, as well as T1-weighted images with different MRI field strengths. The multi-modal set consists of pairs of T1- and T2-weighted images. Dice overlap and HdDist95 (95% quantile of Hausdorff distance) are based on segmentations of over 100 anatomical structures, whereas TRE (target registration error) is based on manual landmarks.

Using MIND features as input representation causes only a very minor drop in in-domain and out-of-domain performance while significantly improving multi-modal performance. The additional strategies systematically improve the performance, although the improvements are not very large. It is noteworthy that the clearly larger non-diffeomorphic volume (NDV) in the baseline version compared to the ones using the MIND feature representation is explained by the multi-modal pairs for which the model predicts very unrealistic deformations.

Table 1. Results showcasing the effects of the proposed design choices on the validation set. The values and metrics are directly from the LUMIR 2025 challenge leaderboard (the method holds the 1st place 2 weeks before the challenge test submission is closed). Please refer to Sect. 4 and the challenge for more details on the metrics. MIND: Transform the input images using the MIND transformation. NDV: Use loss penalizing non-diffeomorphic volume. GC: Use group-consistency loss over image triplets. AUG: Augment input images. ENS: Use ensemble of 5 models.

MIND	NDV	GC	AUG	ENS	Dice(%) ↑			TRE ↓	HdDist95 ↓	NDV ↓
					In-domain	Out-of-domain	Multi-modal	In-domain	Overall	Overall
×	×	×	×	×	77.7(1.5)	76.2(1.5)	28.4(1.5)	2.30(0.32)	4.62(1.88)	0.052(0.042)
✓	×	×	×	×	77.6(1.4)	75.9(1.2)	73.3(2.8)	2.31(0.30)	3.18(0.30)	0.015(0.0022)
✓	✓	✓	×	×	78.0(1.5)	76.0(1.5)	73.7(2.8)	2.27(0.26)	3.02(0.36)	0.0017(3.2e−4)
✓	✓	✓	✓	×	78.0(1.7)	76.2(1.1)	74.2(2.9)	2.26(0.25)	2.99(0.33)	0.0025(4.2e−4)
✓	✓	✓	✓	✓	**78.3**(1.7)	**76.5**(1.2)	**74.5**(3.0)	**2.24**(0.27)	**2.95**(0.34)	**0.0015**(3.3e−4)

5 Discussion

The paper proposes a simple deep learning strategy that allows registration of T1 and T2 weighted MRI scans while training only on T1-weighted MRI scans by transforming the inputs with the MIND transformation before feeding them into the network. Good results indicate that the MIND transformation transforms T1- and T2-weighted MRI images into relatively similar representations. The performance of T1-T2 registration with the proposed method, while close, is still worse than the in-domain performance. A potential future research direction is hence to look for even more suitable input transformations. Further research is also needed on the performance of the method on other modalities or anatomies.

Acknowledgments. This work was supported by the Research Council of Finland (Flagship programme: Finnish Center for Artificial Intelligence FCAI, and grants 352986, 358246) and EU (H2020 grant 101016775 and NextGenerationEU). We also acknowledge the computational resources provided by the Aalto Science-IT Project.

Disclosure of Interests. The authors have no competing interests to declare that are relevant to the content of this article.

References

1. Chen, J., Frey, E.C., He, Y., Segars, W.P., Li, Y., Du, Y.: TransMorph: transformer for unsupervised medical image registration. Med. Image Anal. **82**, 102615 (2022)

2. Dufumier, B., Grigis, A., Victor, J., Ambroise, C., Frouin, V., Duchesnay, E.: OpenBHB: a large-scale multi-site brain MRI data-set for age prediction and debiasing. Neuroimage **263**, 119637 (2022)
3. Gu, D., et al.: Pair-wise and group-wise deformation consistency in deep registration network. In: Martel, A.L., et al. (eds.) MICCAI 2020. LNCS, vol. 12263, pp. 171–180. Springer, Cham (2020). https://doi.org/10.1007/978-3-030-59716-0_17
4. Guo, C.K.: Multi-modal image registration with unsupervised deep learning. Ph.D. thesis, Massachusetts Institute of Technology (2019)
5. Heinrich, M.P., et al.: MIND: modality independent neighbourhood descriptor for multi-modal deformable registration. Med. Image Anal. **16**(7), 1423–1435 (2012)
6. Hering, A., et al.: Learn2Reg: comprehensive multi-task medical image registration challenge, dataset and evaluation in the era of deep learning. IEEE Trans. Med. Imag. **42**(3), 697–712 (2022)
7. Honkamaa, J., Marttinen, P.: SITReg: multi-resolution architecture for symmetric, inverse consistent, and topology preserving image registration. arXiv preprint arXiv:2303.10211 (2023)
8. Jena, R., Sethi, D., Chaudhari, P., Gee, J.: Deep learning in medical image registration: magic or mirage? Adv. Neural. Inf. Process. Syst. **37**, 108331–108353 (2024)
9. Liu, Y., Chen, J., Wei, S., Carass, A., Prince, J.: On finite difference Jacobian computation in deformable image registration. Int. J. Comput. Vision **132**(9), 3678–3688 (2024)
10. Taha, A., et al.: Magnetic resonance imaging datasets with anatomical fiducials for quality control and registration. Sci. Data **10**(1), 449 (2023)

Unleashing the Power of Intensity Augmentation for Multi-modal Image Registration

Bailiang Jian[1,2,3(✉)], Daniel Scholz[1,2,3], Jiazhen Pan[1,2], Morteza Ghahremani[1,2,3], Christian Wachinger[1,2,3], and Benedikt Wiestler[1,2,3]

[1] Technical University of Munich, Munich, Germany
[2] Klinikum Rechts der Isar, Munich, Germany
bailiang.jian@tum.de
[3] Munich Center for Machine Learning, Munich, Germany

Abstract. A key challenge for multi-modal brain MRI registration is that most training data consists of only T1-weighted scans, making it difficult to generalize to other less frequently acquired modalities. We show that purely randomized intensity augmentations, without any annotations or modality synthesis, transform T1-trained networks from complete failure to state-of-the-art performance in T1—T2-weighted registration. Further, enforcing transformation composition consistency across image triplets yields substantial accuracy gains. Together, these simple yet powerful strategies redefine how robust multi-modal registration can be achieved under minimal supervision and data assumptions.

Keywords: Intensity Augmentation · Multi-modal Image Registration

1 Introduction

Multi-modal image registration is a cornerstone of clinical brain analysis, as different MRI modalities emphasize complementary tissue properties. For example, T1-weighted scans provide excellent anatomical detail, T2/FLAIR highlight pathologies such as tumors, edema, or demyelinating lesions, while functional MRI captures brain activation patterns. By spatially aligning these modalities into a common space, clinicians can integrate diverse sources of information for more accurate diagnosis and disease characterization.

Despite its importance, robust multi-modal registration remains a challenging task. Recent modality-agnostic approaches either (i) synthesize images from segmentation labels [3,8], which requires extra annotation efforts and is inherently affected by noise or errors in anatomical segmentations, or (ii) rely on training with large-scale multi-modal datasets [4,23], which is impractical in real clinical settings where T1-weighted MRI is by far the most common modality.

C. Wachinger and B. Wiestler—Equal Advising.

J. Chen et al. (Eds.): Learn2Reg 2025, LNCS 16254, pp. 43–51, 2026.
https://doi.org/10.1007/978-3-032-25169-5_6

To address these limitations, we propose a framework that generalizes a registration network trained solely on T1-weighted MRIs to unseen modalities such as T2-weighted. Our approach is simple, annotation-free, and does not assume access to large multi-modal datasets.

Our key contributions are:

- **Randomized intensity augmentation.** We introduce a set of purely randomized intensity transformations that simulate diverse modality appearances. These augmentations enable the network to perform accurate T1–T2-weighted registration, where baseline models completely fail.
- **Transformation composition consistency.** We adapt the longitudinal transformation composition consistency [10] to the cross-sectional setting. Enforcing consistency across composed transformations significantly improves registration accuracy and robustness, leading to large gains in accuracy metrics.

2 Methodology

2.1 Registration Network

As demonstrated in [9], registration-specific design choices are often more critical than sophisticated computational blocks. Therefore, we adopt the "DWCPI" variant proposed in [9], which emphasizes five essential components: **D**ual-stream encoding, **W**arping, **C**orrelation, **P**yramidal decoders, and **I**terative refinement (Fig. 1).

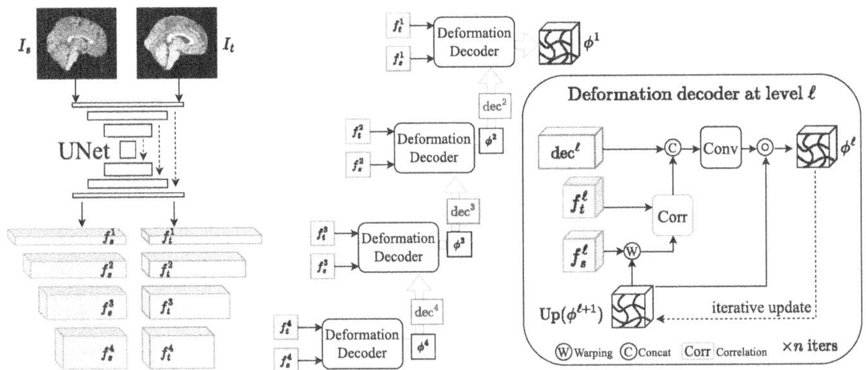

Fig. 1. Overview of the registration network architecture. The source image I_s and target image I_t are encoded by a UNet encoder (***Dual-stream encoding***), generating two sets of pyramidal feature maps. The pyramidal deformation decoders then predict deformation fields at each resolution level ℓ, where level ℓ corresponds to $2^{-\ell}$ resolution. Within each decoder, registration-specific components (***Warping***, ***Correlation***, and ***Iteration***) are applied.

Dual-Stream Encoder (D). We extract feature maps from both source (I_s) and target (I_t) images via weight-sharing encoder. At each resolution level ℓ ($2^{-\ell}$ resolution), the encoder produces pyramidal features f_s^ℓ and f_t^ℓ, with $\ell = 4, 3, 2, 1$ denoting increasing spatial resolution.

Warping (W) and Pyramidal Decoders (P). Deformation is predicted in a coarse-to-fine manner. At each level ℓ, the source feature map f_s^ℓ is first warped using the upsampled and upscaled deformation field $\mathrm{Up}(\phi^{\ell+1})$ estimated from the previous coarser level:

$$\tilde{f}_s^\ell = f_s^\ell \circ \mathrm{Up}(\phi^{\ell+1}).$$

The warped source feature $\tilde{f}_s^\ell$ and target feature f_t^ℓ are then passed to the correlation layer for local similarity computation.

Correlation (C). To guide deformation estimation, we compute local correlation volumes between $\tilde{f}_s^\ell$ and f_t^ℓ. Specifically, let $\mathbf{f}_t, \mathbf{f}_s \in \mathbb{R}^{H \times W \times D \times N}$ be the feature maps, with N the channel dimension. For each voxel $p = (x, y, z)$ in $\mathbf{f}_t$, we compute correlations with source features in a local neighborhood $\mathcal{N}_d(p)$ of radius d:

$$\mathbf{C}(p, \Delta) = \frac{1}{N} \mathbf{f}_t(p)^\top \mathbf{f}_s(p + \Delta), \quad \Delta \in \mathcal{N}_d(p),$$

resulting in a correlation volume $\mathbf{C} \in \mathbb{R}^{H \times W \times D \times (2d+1)^3}$. This localized formulation significantly reduces the computational cost compared to full all-to-all correlations [6,11,16,22].

Iterative Refinement (I). Finally, at each resolution level ℓ, the decoder performs multiple iterations of correlation computation and flow update [14,17, 18,22,25]. This iterative process progressively refines the predicted deformation ϕ^ℓ, before passing it to the next finer level.

U-Net Backbone Encoder (U). Instead of the single contracting encoder used in [9], we employ a full U-Net backbone. This leverages the decoding path to forward richer multi-scale features [5,13].

2.2 Randomized Intensity Augmentation

To improve robustness to unseen modalities and domain shifts, we employ a set of randomized intensity augmentations that perturb image appearance while preserving anatomical structure. These augmentations expose the network to diverse intensity distributions, enabling it to generalize from T1-weighted MRI training data to other modalities such as T2-weighted or FLAIR (Fig. 2).

Random Convolution. We apply randomly initialized convolutional filters to the input image [15,19,24], which alters local intensity patterns and edge responses. This simulates different imaging contrasts and acquisition settings, encouraging the registration network to be modality-agnostic.

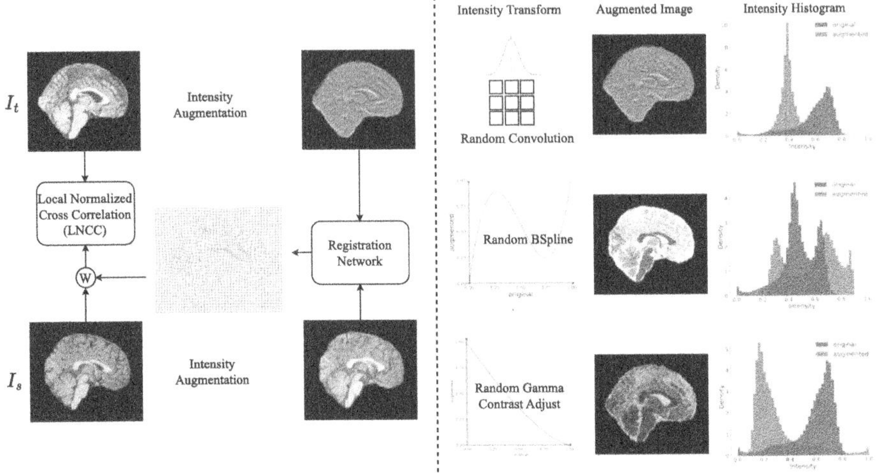

Fig. 2. Left: Training workflow. Intensity augmentations are applied to T1-weighted images before being input into the registration network. The predicted deformation field warps the original T1-weighted source image, and mono-modal image similarity (LNCC) is computed between the warped and target T1-weighted images. **Right**: Examples of intensity augmentation methods, including *random convolution*, *random B-spline transformation*, and *random gamma contrast adjustment*.

Random B-Spline Intensity Transform. A cubic B-spline is fit over the image intensity range with randomly sampled knot values. This defines a smooth nonlinear mapping of voxel intensities, optionally inverted with a given probability. The transform perturbs global and local contrast in a controlled yet randomized fashion, approximating the appearance variations between MRI modalities.

Random Gamma Contrast Adjustment. We randomly sample a gamma value and apply a gamma-power transformation to the normalized image intensities, optionally with inversion. This operation modifies the intensity distribution by emphasizing bright or dark regions, simulating scanner- or protocol-dependent contrast differences.

Random Bias Field. To further account for domain-specific acquisition artifacts, we simulate spatially varying intensity inhomogeneities by applying a random bias field. This encourages the network to become robust to coil sensitivity variations and scanner-dependent shading artifacts.

Together, these randomized augmentations generate a diverse set of intensity distributions without requiring additional annotated data, substantially enhancing the registration network's ability to generalize across modalities and domains (Fig. 3).

2.3 Tranformation Composition Consistency

Transformation consistency is a fundamental property of spatial mappings: composing deformations $I_0 \to I_1$ and $I_1 \to I_2$ should yield a deformation consistent with the direct mapping $I_0 \to I_2$. Inspired by longitudinal consistency losses [10], we adapt this idea to the cross-sectional setting.

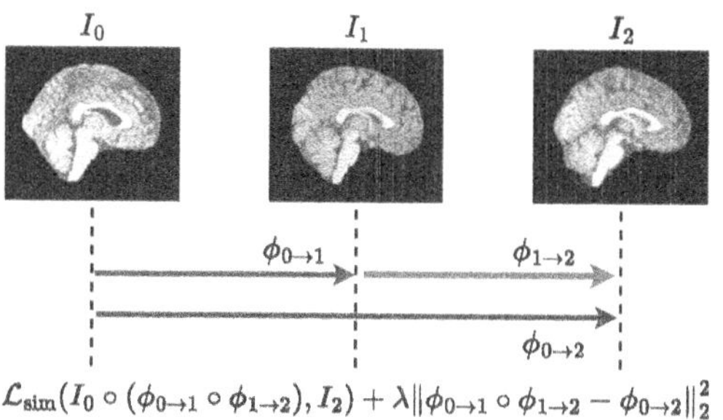

Fig. 3. Overview of the transformation composition consistency loss. Pairwise registrations are performed between I_0 and I_1, I_1 and I_2, and I_0 and I_2, producing deformation fields $\phi_{0\to1}$, $\phi_{1\to2}$, and $\phi_{0\to2}$. Image similarity is computed between I_2 and I_0 warped by the composition $\phi_{0\to1} \circ \phi_{1\to2}$. The ℓ_2 distance between $\phi_{0\to1} \circ \phi_{1\to2}$ and $\phi_{0\to2}$ enforces consistency of the deformation fields under transformation composition.

Given a triplet of images (I_0, I_1, I_2) randomly sampled from the training dataset (effectively acting as a batch of size 3), we perform pairwise registrations to estimate $\phi_{0\to1}$, $\phi_{1\to2}$, and $\phi_{0\to2}$. We then define the transformation composition consistency loss as

$$\mathcal{L}_{\text{TCC}} = \mathcal{L}_{\text{sim}}\big(I_0 \circ (\phi_{0\to1} \circ \phi_{1\to2}),\, I_2\big) + \lambda\, \|\phi_{0\to2} - (\phi_{0\to1} \circ \phi_{1\to2})\|_2^2, \tag{1}$$

where the first term enforces image similarity between the composed warp of I_0 and the target I_2, and the second term explicitly penalizes discrepancies between the composed deformation and the direct deformation $\phi_{0\to2}$.

This formulation provides additional supervision beyond standard pairwise training: when the network registers $I_0 \leftrightarrow I_1$ and $I_1 \leftrightarrow I_2$, it is simultaneously guided to maintain transitivity across the triplet. This formulation can be naturally extended to $N > 3$ images by enforcing consistency between the direct transformation $\phi_{0\to N-1}$ and the composed chain $\phi_{0\to1} \circ \cdots \circ \phi_{N-2\to N-1}$. In practice, this synergy substantially improves registration accuracy.

3 Experiments and Results

To assess the proposed method, we conduct both offline and online evaluations on the LUMIR [2,7,21] validation set.[1] For the offline evaluation, segmentation

[1] https://learn2reg.grand-challenge.org/#lumir-2025.

labels are generated using SynthSeg [1]. Registration accuracy is measured by the Dice score between the warped source labels and the target labels, while deformation field regularity is quantified by the non-diffeomorphic voxels (NDV) [12]. For the online evaluation, metric numbers are retrieved from the LUMIR25 leaderboard[2].

Table 1. Offline evaluation on the LUMIR validation set. Results are reported for in-distribution (ID), out-of-distribution (OOD), and multi-modal (MM, T1–T2-weighted) registration. Dice score (DSC) measures registration accuracy, and non-diffeomorphic voxels with the foreground brain area (NDV in scale of 10^{-4}) quantify deformation regularity. TCC denotes the proposed Transformation Composition Consistency loss.

	ID		OOD		MM	
	DSC ↑	NDV(‱) ↓	DSC ↑	NDV(‱) ↓	DSC ↑	NDV(‱) ↓
initial	63.59 ± 3.89	–	60.84 ± 4.28	–	64.29 ± 4.49	–
UDWCPI	85.37 ± 1.60	0.81 ± 0.28	83.46 ± 3.02	0.52 ± 0.37	25.12 ± 3.08	0.80 ± 0.15
+aug	84.37 ± 1.35	0.61 ± 0.23	82.72 ± 2.71	0.35 ± 0.35	81.37 ± 1.11	0.13 ± 0.03
+aug+TCC	86.05 ± 1.46	4.38 ± 1.35	84.77 ± 2.48	2.53 ± 0.26	83.00 ± 0.86	2.88 ± 0.70

Table 2. Online evaluation results on the LUMIR25 validation leaderboard. Results are reported for in-distribution (ID), out-of-distribution (OOD), and multi-modal (MM, T1–T2-weighted) registration. Accuracy is measured by Dice score (DSC), 95th percentile Hausdorff distance (HD95), and target registration error (TRE). Deformation regularity is quantified by the non-diffeomorphic volume (NDV). Mean values are presented.

	ID		OOD			MM		NDV ↓
	DSC ↑	HD95 ↓	DSC ↑	HD95 ↓	TRE ↓	DSC ↑	HD95 ↓	
initial	56.68	4.79	51.89	5.27	4.35	53.91	4.38	–
ConvexAdam	69.98	3.83	66.21	4.01	2.51	65.78	3.46	10^{-3}
SynthMorph	72.62	3.58	68.88	3.91	2.61	68.88	3.25	10^{-5}
VFA+SynSR	77.44	3.20	75.45	3.30	2.50	73.20	2.82	7×10^{-3}
no-aug+TCC	78.08	3.11	76.15	3.22	2.31	41.19	5.60	0.3
aug+TCC	77.96	3.11	76.06	3.22	2.32	74.22	2.64	0.08
final	78.17	3.09	76.11	3.19	2.32	74.44	2.60	0.017

[2] https://learn2reg.grand-challenge.org/evaluation/l2r25-lumir25/leaderboard/.

Offline Evaluation. As shown in Table 1, randomized intensity augmentation enables a significant improvement in multi-modal registration: the DSC increases from a failed baseline of 25.12 to 81.37. Adding Transformation Composition Consistency (TCC) provides a further boost across all settings. Although NDV values increase when TCC is applied, the absolute ratios remain very low (on the order of 3×10^{-4}), indicating that deformation fields are still smooth. Building on these results, we further finetune the method by adding an explicit penalty on the number of voxels with non-positive Jacobian determinants to better satisfy the smoothness constraints (Fig. 4).

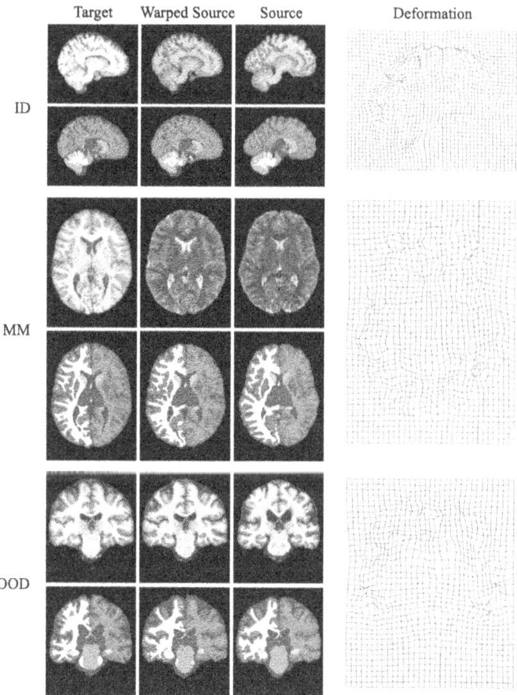

Fig. 4. Qualitative results of the submitted solution. The source, target, and warped source images/segmentation labels together with deformation fields are presented for in-distribution (ID), out-of-distribution (OOD), and multi-modal (MM) T1-T2-weighted registration.

Online Evaluation. In Table 2, we report the online evaluation results retrieved from the LUMIR25 validation leaderboard. Among the baselines, ConvexAdam [20] and SynthMorph [8] are modality-agnostic approaches, yet they achieve only moderate performance. VFA [13] combined with SynthSR, which synthesizes T1-weighted MRI from T2-weighted and thereby reduces the multi-modal task to mono-modal registration, achieves strong results. Consistent with our offline evaluation, our method without augmentation completely fails in the multi-modal (T1—T2-weighted) setting. However, once augmented with randomized intensity transforms, our approach achieves the best multi-modal performance, surpassing all baselines while maintaining competitive accuracy in both ID and OOD scenarios.

4 Discussion

Our experiments demonstrate that randomized intensity augmentation is a powerful strategy for bridging the modality gap in brain MRI registration. By exposing the network to diverse synthetic intensity distributions, we achieve robust generalization from T1-only training to T2-weighted registration, effectively transforming a failed baseline into strong multi-modal performance. Complementing this, the proposed transformation composition consistency loss provides additional structural supervision, yielding consistent gains in registration accuracy. These results suggest that simple, annotation-free augmentations coupled with transitivity consistency constraints can substantially improve the practicality of learning-based registration.

Acknowledgments. This work was supported by BMWi (project "NeuroTEMP") research funding and the Munich Center of Machine Learning (MCML).

References

1. Billot, B., Iglesias, J.E., et al.: SynthSeg: segmentation of brain MRI scans of any contrast and resolution without retraining. Med. Image Anal. **86**, 102789 (2023)
2. Chen, J., et al.: Beyond the LUMIR challenge: the pathway to foundational registration models. arXiv preprint arXiv:2505.24160 (2025)
3. Chen, J., Wei, S., Liu, Y., Carass, A., Du, Y.: Pretraining deformable image registration networks with random images. In: Medical Imaging with Deep Learning-Short Papers (2025)
4. Demir, B., et al.: multiGradICON: a foundation model for multimodal medical image registration. In: International Workshop on Biomedical Image Registration, pp. 3–18. Springer (2024)
5. Dey, N., et al.: Learning general-purpose biomedical volume representations using randomized synthesis. In: The Thirteenth International Conference on Learning Representations (2025)
6. Dosovitskiy, A., Fischer, P., Ilg, E., et al.: FlowNet: learning optical flow with convolutional networks. In: Proceedings of the IEEE International Conference on Computer Vision, pp. 2758–2766 (2015)
7. Dufumier, B., Grigis, A., Victor, J., Ambroise, C., Frouin, V., Duchesnay, E.: OpenBHB: a large-scale multi-site brain MRI data-set for age prediction and debiasing. Neuroimage **263**, 119637 (2022)
8. Hoffmann, M., Hoopes, A., Greve, D.N., Fischl, B., Dalca, A.V.: Anatomy-aware and acquisition-agnostic joint registration with SynthMorph. Imaging Neurosci. **2**, 1–33 (2024)

9. Jian, B., Pan, J., Ghahremani, M., Rueckert, D., Wachinger, C., Wiestler, B.: Mamba? Catch the hype or rethink what really helps for image registration. In: International Workshop on Biomedical Image Registration, pp. 86–97. Springer (2024)
10. Jian, B., et al.: TimeFlow: longitudinal brain image registration and aging progression analysis. arXiv preprint arXiv:2501.08667 (2025)
11. Kang, M., Hu, X., Huang, W., et al.: Dual-stream pyramid registration network. Med. Image Anal. **78**, 102379 (2022)
12. Liu, Y., Chen, J., Wei, S., Carass, A., Prince, J.: On finite difference Jacobian computation in deformable image registration. Int. J. Comput. Vis., 1–11 (2024)
13. Liu, Y., Chen, J., Zuo, L., Carass, A., Prince, J.L.: Vector field attention for deformable image registration. J. Med. Imag. **11**(6), 064001 (2024)
14. Ma, T., Zhang, S., Li, J., Wen, Y.: IIRP-Net: iterative inference residual pyramid network for enhanced image registration. In: Proceedings of the IEEE/CVF Conference on Computer Vision and Pattern Recognition, pp. 11546–11555 (2024)
15. Ouyang, C., et al.: Causality-inspired single-source domain generalization for medical image segmentation. IEEE Trans. Med. Imaging **42**(4), 1095–1106 (2022)
16. Pan, J., Huang, W., Rueckert, D., Küstner, T., Hammernik, K.: Reconstruction-driven motion estimation for motion-compensated MR CINE imaging. IEEE Trans. Med. Imag. (2024)
17. Pan, J., Rueckert, D., Küstner, T., Hammernik, K.: Efficient image registration network for non-rigid cardiac motion estimation. In: Haq, N., Johnson, P., Maier, A., Würfl, T., Yoo, J. (eds.) MLMIR 2021. LNCS, vol. 12964, pp. 14–24. Springer, Cham (2021). https://doi.org/10.1007/978-3-030-88552-6_2
18. Qiu, H., Hammernik, K., Qin, C., Chen, C., Rueckert, D.: Embedding gradient-based optimization in image registration networks. In: International Conference on Medical Image Computing and Computer-Assisted Intervention, pp. 56–65. Springer (2022)
19. Sideri-Lampretsa, V., Zimmer, V.A., Qiu, H., Kaissis, G., Rueckert, D.: MAD: modality agnostic distance measure for image registration. In: International Conference on Medical Image Computing and Computer-Assisted Intervention, pp. 147–156. Springer (2023)
20. Siebert, H., Großbröhmer, C., Hansen, L., Heinrich, M.P.: ConvexAdam: self-configuring dual-optimisation-based 3D multitask medical image registration. IEEE Trans. Med. Imag. (2024)
21. Taha, A., et al.: Magnetic resonance imaging datasets with anatomical fiducials for quality control and registration. Sci. Data **10**(1), 449 (2023)
22. Teed, Z., Deng, J.: RAFT: recurrent all-pairs field transforms for optical flow. In: Vedaldi, A., Bischof, H., Brox, T., Frahm, J.-M. (eds.) ECCV 2020. LNCS, vol. 12347, pp. 402–419. Springer, Cham (2020). https://doi.org/10.1007/978-3-030-58536-5_24
23. Tian, L., et al.: uniGradICON: a foundation model for medical image registration. In: International Conference on Medical Image Computing and Computer-Assisted Intervention, pp. 749–760. Springer (2024)
24. Xu, Z., Liu, D., Yang, J., Raffel, C., Niethammer, M.: Robust and generalizable visual representation learning via random convolutions. arXiv preprint arXiv:2007.13003 (2020)
25. Zhao, S., Dong, Y., Chang, E.I., Xu, Y., et al.: Recursive cascaded networks for unsupervised medical image registration. In: Proceedings of the IEEE/CVF International Conference on Computer Vision, pp. 10600–10610 (2019)

Adapting Frozen Mono-modal Backbones for Multi-Modal Registration via Contrast-Agnostic Instance Optimization

Yi Zhang, Yidong Zhao, and Qian Tao(✉)

Department of Imaging Physics, Delft University of Technology, Delft, The Netherlands
q.tao@tudelft.nl

Abstract. Deformable image registration remains a central challenge in medical image analysis, particularly under multi-modal scenarios where intensity distributions vary significantly across scans. While deep learning methods provide efficient feed-forward predictions, they often fail to generalize robustly under distribution shifts at test time. A straightforward remedy is full network fine-tuning, yet for modern architectures such as Transformers or deep U-Nets, this adaptation is prohibitively expensive in both memory and runtime when operating in 3D. Meanwhile, the naive fine-tuning struggles more with potential degradation in performance in the existence of drastic domain shifts. In this work, we propose a registration framework that integrates a frozen pretrained **mono-modal** registration model with a lightweight adaptation pipeline for **multi-modal** image registration. Specifically, we employ style transfer based on contrast-agnostic representation generation and refinement modules to bridge modality and domain gaps with instance optimization at test time. This design is orthogonal to the choice of backbone mono-modal model, thus avoids the computational burden of full fine-tuning while retaining the flexibility to adapt to unseen domains. We evaluate our approach on the Learn2Reg 2025 LUMIR validation set and observe consistent improvements over the pretrained state-of-the-art mono-modal backbone. In particular, the method ranks second on the multi-modal subset, third on the out-of-domain subset, and achieves fourth place overall in Dice score. These results demonstrate that combining frozen mono-modal models with modality adaptation and lightweight instance optimization offers an effective and practical pathway toward robust multi-modal registration.

Keywords: Deformable image registration · Multi-modal image analysis · Contrast-agnostic representations

---

This paper was prepared as part of the Learn2Reg Challenge of MICCAI 2025.

J. Chen et al. (Eds.): Learn2Reg 2025, LNCS 16254, pp. 52–61, 2026.
https://doi.org/10.1007/978-3-032-25169-5_7

1 Introduction

Medical image registration establishes anatomical correspondences between medical images and remains a prerequisite for applications such as treatment planning and longitudinal studies [12,25,26]. Classical approaches optimize a similarity-regularization objective with respect to a parameterized transformation for each image pair [13]. Recent advances in machine learning have reshaped medical image registration by replacing per-case optimization with data-driven prediction [23]. Unsupervised frameworks typically retain the classical objective which still combines an image similarity term with deformation regularization but optimize it through neural networks trained across many pairs in a population [1,5]. Since the advent of U-Net [22], a rich family of unsupervised registration architectures has emerged [1,4]. More recently, alternative backbones such as Transformers [2], implicit neural representations [8,30], and dual encoders [16] have been explored to capture long-range dependencies and continuous deformation fields.

A persistent challenge is *cross-modality* registration, where varying MRI contrasts (*e.g.*, T1w, T2w, FLAIR) disrupt simple intensity correspondences. This issue has been emphasized in the 2025 Learn2Reg LUMIR track, which evaluates robustness under contrast shifts and zero-shot settings [3,7,17,27]. Classical cross-modality registration often employs mutual information (MI) and its variants [29], or modality-agnostic local descriptors such as MIND [9]. Learning-based strategies include deep metric learning for multi-modal similarity [18,20], image-to-image translation to synthesize target-like contrast [21], and contrast-invariant training regimes [10]. Despite these advances, modern pretrained backbones still suffer substantial performance drops when tested outside their native mono-modal domain.

Instance optimization (IO) has emerged as a lightweight means of test-time adaptation by updating parameters for each image pair [1,19,28]. However, full fine-tuning of large 3D models such as U-Nets or Transformers remains prohibitively expensive, and naive IO may be unstable under severe modality gaps. With the recent availability of foundational registration backbones [6,28], the key question is how to adapt these powerful yet mono-modal models efficiently to multi-modal or out-of-domain scenarios.

In this work, we introduce a contrast-agnostic instance optimization framework that acts as a general test-time adaptor for pretrained registration backbones. By taking the backbone output as initialization and applying a gated style-transfer module with lightweight refinement, the method remains orthogonal to backbone choice and incurs minor overhead. Beyond improving cross-modality robustness, it consistently enhances in-domain performance of state-of-the-art mono-modal baselines. Validated on the Learn2Reg 2025 LUMIR benchmark, our approach demonstrates competitive accuracy across in-domain, out-of-domain, and multi-modal tracks, establishing a lightweight and broadly applicable adaptor for robust multi-modal deformable registration.

2 Methods

2.1 Deformable Image Registration

Given a pair of 3D images $I_{\mathrm{A}} \in \mathbb{R}^{D\times H\times W}$ and $I_{\mathrm{B}} \in \mathbb{R}^{D\times H\times W}$, deformable registration seeks a dense transformation $\phi \in \mathbb{R}^{3\times D\times H\times W}$ such that the warped source $I_{\mathrm{A}} \circ \phi$ is anatomically aligned to the target I_{B}. As the deformation is typically small relative to the image grid x, it is expressed as $\phi(x) = x + u(x)$ with a displacement field u. The registration task can be formulated as the optimization

$$\hat{\phi} = \underset{\phi}{\operatorname{argmin}}\ \mathcal{L}_{\mathrm{sim}}(I_{\mathrm{A}} \circ \phi, I_{\mathrm{B}}) + \lambda \mathcal{L}_{\mathrm{reg}}(\phi), \tag{1}$$

where $\mathcal{L}_{\mathrm{sim}}$ measures image similarity and $\mathcal{L}_{\mathrm{reg}}$ regularizes the deformation field with trade-off parameter $\lambda > 0$ (Fig. 1).

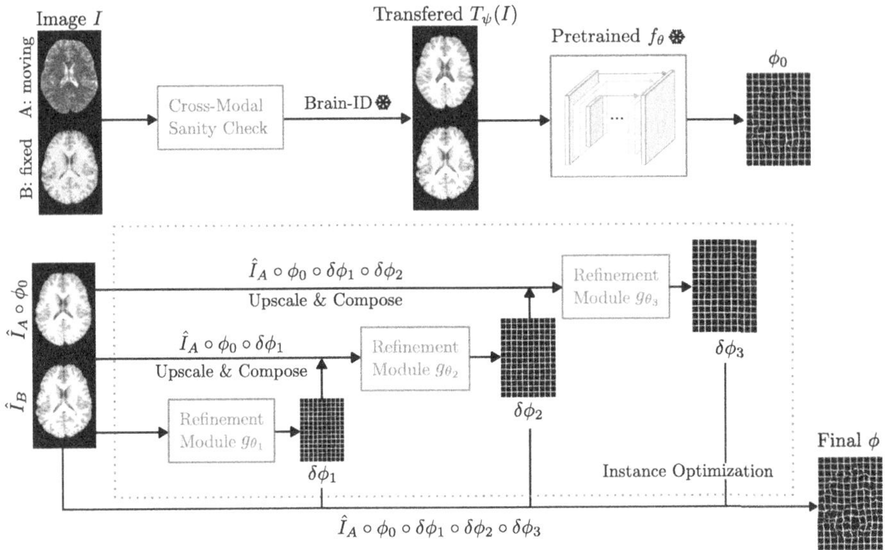

Fig. 1. Overview of the proposed framework. Input images are optionally passed through a contrast-agnostic preprocessing (Brain-ID) when large modality differences are detected. A frozen pretrained backbone f_θ produces an initialization ϕ_0, which is refined by instance optimization with lightweight multi-scale modules. The final deformation field ϕ_T is obtained by composing these refinements.

2.2 Instance Optimization Formulation

Let f_θ denote the backbone network, pretrained on a mono-modal dataset. For each image pair (I_A, I_B), the initial deformation field is estimated as

$$\phi_0 = f_\theta(I_A, I_B). \tag{2}$$

However, due to distribution shifts, this initialization can be suboptimal. Several refinement strategies have been considered in the literature: (1) iterative application of f_θ by feeding the warped source $I_A \circ \phi_0$ as the new input; (2) direct optimization of the backbone parameters under the objective in Eq. 1 [28]; and (3) employing ϕ_0 as an initialization for a subsequent registration stage, in analogy to classical sequential pipelines (e.g., affine initialization followed by deformable refinement).

Previous studies have reported that repeated application of a one-step network (e.g. VoxelMorph) leads to cumulative propagation of errors and poor accuracy [31]. Moreover, strategy (2) entails prohibitively high computational requirements: a single forward–backward pass already exceeds 24 GB of VRAM for models with attention mechanism, rendering fine-tuning infeasible on widely accessible GPUs.

Therefore, we adopt the third strategy: using ϕ_0 and $I_A \circ \phi_0$ as initialization for a lightweight refinement stage. In this way, the pretrained backbone remains frozen, avoiding the cost of fine-tuning while still benefiting from its strong initialization. Since the refinement only acts on the output field, the approach is naturally orthogonal to the choice of backbone.

2.3 Progressive Refinement Network

Given the initial deformation $\phi_0 = f_\theta(I_A, I_B)$, we introduce a cascaded refinement module composed of three randomly initialized 3D U-Nets $\{g_{\theta_1}, g_{\theta_2}, g_{\theta_3}\}$. Each network predicts a residual deformation at progressively finer scales.

At stage $t \in \{1, 2, 3\}$, the current warped source $I_A \circ \phi_{t-1}$ together with the target I_B is passed to g_{θ_t} to estimate a residual field $\delta\phi_t$ at a reduced resolution s_t:

$$\delta\phi_t = g_{\theta_t}(I_A \circ \phi_{t-1}, I_B), \quad s_t \in \left\{\tfrac{1}{4}, \tfrac{1}{2}, 1\right\}. \tag{3}$$

This residual is then upsampled to the original resolution and composed with the previous deformation:

$$\phi_t = \phi_{t-1} \circ \text{Upsample}(\delta\phi_t). \tag{4}$$

Recursively, the full refinement process can be summarized as:

$$\phi_T = \phi_0 \circ \prod_{t=1}^{T} \text{Upsample}\big(g_{\theta_t}(I_A \circ \phi_{t-1}, I_B)\big), \quad T = 3, \tag{5}$$

where the product $\prod$ denotes successive composition of the deformation fields. The final field ϕ_T integrates both the pretrained initialization ϕ_0 and the multi-scale residual refinements $\{\delta\phi_1, \delta\phi_2, \delta\phi_3\}$. The refinement admits a brief pre-training to provide more stable initialization, while still avoiding the computational burden of full fine-tuning.

2.4 Contrast-Agnostic Representation via Brain-ID

When the input modality differs substantially from the training domain, the limited steps available for IO can lead to suboptimal adaptation given the inaccurate initialization. To mitigate such distribution gaps, we employ Brain-ID [14], a publicly available model that provides contrast-invariant representations and T1w-like style-transferred images. Given an input I, Brain-ID produces

$$\hat{I} = T_{\psi}(I), \qquad z(I) = R_{\psi}(I), \tag{6}$$

where T_{ψ} is a frozen style-transfer module and R_{ψ} is a contrast-robust encoder. We then use the transferred pair $(\hat{I}_A, \hat{I}_B)$ to compute the backbone initialization

$$\phi_0 = f_{\theta}(\hat{I}_A, \hat{I}_B). \tag{7}$$

Since both T_{ψ} and R_{ψ} are fixed pretrained modules trained on different data, they are not explicitly optimized for f_{θ}. While Brain-ID improves robustness under distribution shifts, it may not preserve all T1w details. Therefore, we apply Brain-ID only when a fast (<0.5 s in deployment) similarity check indicates a modality gap: if the low-resolution LNCC between (I_A, I_B) falls below a threshold τ, the pair is routed through Brain-ID; otherwise, the original images are used.

2.5 Loss Functions

We adopt LNCC with a Gaussian kernel of 9 voxels as the similarity term $\mathcal{L}_{\text{sim}}$. At each refinement stage t, the warped source $I_A \circ \phi_t$ is compared with I_B, and the overall loss combines multi-level similarities with a diffusion regularizer on the final deformation ϕ_T:

$$\mathcal{L} = \sum_{t=1}^{T} \mathcal{L}_{\text{sim}}(I_A \circ \phi_t, I_B) + \lambda \mathcal{L}_{\text{reg}}(\phi_T), \quad T = 3. \tag{8}$$

When Brain-ID is used, (I_A, I_B) are replaced by their transferred counterparts $(\hat{I}_A, \hat{I}_B)$.

3 Experiments

3.1 Data

We conducted our experiments on the 2025 L2R Challenge LUMIR dataset [3,7,17,27], which consists of T1-weighted brain MRI scans from 10 public datasets. The dataset includes 3384 subjects for training, 36 subjects for validation which are available to the participants. All images were resampled and cropped to focus on the region of interest, resulting in an image size of [160, 224, 192].

The validation set contains in-domain, out-of-domain, and multi-modal pairs, and evaluation is conducted on the official platform with Dice score, HD, non-diffeomorphic volume (NDV) [15], and target registration error (TRE) (on the in-domain subset).

3.2 Experimental Settings

We use the public weight of Vector Field Attention (VFA) backbone [16] as f_θ, the official baseline model for LUMIR 2025 challenge pretrained on mono-modal T1-weighted brain MRI. For Brain-ID transfer, we use a LNCC of window size of 11 and $\tau = 0.4$ for modality detection. For the refinement modules, we use a standard U-Net for each module with a base channel counts of 32 and depth of 3 blocks. We use $\lambda = 0.1$ for Eq. 1 with a output magnitude scaling of 0.05 on ϕ_T in the finest resolution to avoid introducing large deformation. For IO, we use Adam optimizer, with a learning rate of 5e−4 and a linear warm up for 10 steps. The number of IO step is set to 50 steps in this work for the compatibility of finishing each pair of registration within 1 min. We pretrained the refinement modules for 1000 steps on the Brain-ID transferred images on the training split for a more stable initialization with Adam optimizer and a learning rate of 1e−5. All experiments except official baselines on the leadboard are implemented on a workstation with NVIDIA RTX5090 with 32G of VRAM with PyTorch 2.8.0. All further implementation details will be included in the public code repository after the test phase evaluation.

We compared our method against both official challenge baselines and several related designs, including: (1) Zero displacement (raw), (2) ConvexAdam-MIND [24], (3) SynthMorph [10], (4) VFA-SynthSR, where SynthSR [11] normalizes inputs to T1w space before VFA, and (5) MultiGradICON (IO) [6] with 50-step IO.

For our proposed pipeline, we also conducted ablation studies on our design choices, resulting in the following variants: (1) Brain-ID replacement (similar to VFA-SynthSR but replacing both inputs when non-T1w images are detected), (2) single U-Net instead of a multi-level cascade, (3) cascaded refinement with additive updates instead of composition, and (4) cascaded refinement with weights initialized from 1000-step pretraining on Brain-ID.

In addition to the leaderboard submissions, we also examined several important baselines on the organizers' reduced 10-class validation set due to the leaderboard submission limit. This includes: (1) VFA with multi-modal pretrained weight on brain MRI, provided by the official repository of LUMIR, (2) VFA-Brain-ID with full finetuning of the network parameters, (3) initializing refinement modules with different pretraining schedules (no pretrain, 1K steps, 5K steps).

4 Results and Discussion

Main Comparison on Validation Leaderboard. Table 1 summarizes the performance of official baselines and our proposed variants on the public validation leaderboard. Compared to VFA-SynthSR, our Brain-ID based pipeline consistently achieves higher Dice on the multi-modal split, confirming the advantage of contrast-agnostic transfer in bridging modality gaps.

Table 1. Performance of official baselines and our variants on the validation leaderboard. Due to space constraints, TRE and HdDist95 are omitted; the full results are available on the official leaderboard.

Method	Overall DICE ↑	NDV (%) ↓	In-domain ↑	Out-of-domain ↑	Multi-modal ↑
Zero Displacement	0.5416 ± 0.0341	–	0.5668	0.5189	0.5391
ConvexAdam-MIND [24]	0.6732 ± 0.0275	0.0010	0.6998	0.6621	0.6578
SynthMorph [10]	0.7012 ± 0.0265	**0.0000**	0.7262	0.6888	0.6888
VFA-SynthSR [11]	0.7536 ± 0.0260	0.0074	0.7744	0.7545	0.7320
MultiGradICON [6]	0.7429 ± 0.0236	0.0017	0.7611	0.7453	0.7222
VFA-Brain-ID (no IO)	0.7563 ± 0.0239	0.0791	0.7743	0.7548	0.7397
VFA-Brain-ID (Single)	0.7569 ± 0.0237	0.0675	0.7747	0.7555	0.7406
VFA-Brain-ID (Add)	0.7580 ± 0.0241	0.0539	0.7744	0.7593	0.7403
VFA-Brain-ID (1K)	$\mathbf{0.7601 \pm 0.0237}$	0.0896	**0.7756**	**0.7617**	**0.7430**

The variants results in Table 1 further highlight the importance of our architectural design. Multi-level cascaded refinement with compositional updates yields noticable gains over both the single-network and additive alternatives, while moderate pretraining (1K steps) provides the best overall Dice. These results suggest that lightweight refinement can effectively adapt frozen backbones without costly full-model tuning. In terms of efficiency, the entire refinement stage requires less than 10 GB GPU memory, making it substantially lighter than fine-tuning modern large 3D backbones.

Table 2. Local validation results on the organizers' reduced 10-class label set. Note that these results are for development only and may not perfectly correlate with the official leaderboard metrics.

Method	Overall DSC ↑	In-domain ↑	Out-of-domain ↑	Multi-modal ↑
VFA Multi-modal (w/o IO)	0.8874 ± 0.0182	0.9001 ± 0.0085	0.8828 ± 0.0195	0.8837 ± 0.0187
VFA-Brain-ID (w/o IO)	0.8896 ± 0.0180	0.9017 ± 0.0088	0.8896 ± 0.0187	0.8830 ± 0.0190
VFA-Brain-ID (full finetune)	0.8863 ± 0.0188	0.8990 ± 0.0079	0.8817 ± 0.0204	0.8820 ± 0.0200
VFA-Brain-ID (w/o pretrain)	0.8930 ± 0.0184	0.9057 ± 0.0086	0.8941 ± 0.0200	0.8857 ± 0.0181
VFA-Brain-ID (1K)	$\mathbf{0.8938 \pm 0.0180}$	$\mathbf{0.9068 \pm 0.0072}$	$\mathbf{0.8945 \pm 0.0200}$	$\mathbf{0.8861 \pm 0.0178}$
VFA-Brain-ID (5K)	0.8929 ± 0.0181	0.9048 ± 0.0074	0.8933 ± 0.0205	0.8861 ± 0.0180

Additional Ablation Studies on Local Validation Subset. Table 2 reports additional ablations on the reduced 10-class validation set. The official multi-modal pretrained VFA achieves strong Dice on the multi-modal subset, but its in-domain and out-of-domain performance are inferior to our Brain-ID adaptor with similarity check, suggesting that contrast-agnostic test-time adaptation generalizes more reliably. Full finetuning of the VFA backbone performs worse than baseline without IO across all subsets, confirming that lightweight adaptation is more robust than exhaustive retraining of the whole model in this case. Finally, we observe that moderate pretraining of the refinement modules (1000 steps) yields the best overall Dice and out-of-domain accuracy, while longer adaptation (5000 steps) provides no additional gains and even slight degradation. These findings indicate that while limited pretraining can stabilize IO, excessive adaptation leads to diminishing returns. We emphasize that these findings are based on the reduced-label validation and should be considered indicative rather than definitive, as they may not fully correlate with the official leaderboard metrics.

IO Dynamics *w.r.t.* Losses and Dice Scores. Figure 2 illustrates the dynamics of instance optimization on the reduced 10-class validation set. On average, IO consistently improves both similarity loss and Dice, confirming that lightweight test-time adaptation can provide measurable gains even with frozen backbones. With a small regularization weight ($\lambda = 0.1$), foldings increase slightly but remain mild given the low initial rate. Although case-wise Dice trajectories are variable and some instances exhibit small drops, such fluctuations are expected in a fully unsupervised setting and highlight opportunities for future refinement of IO strategies.

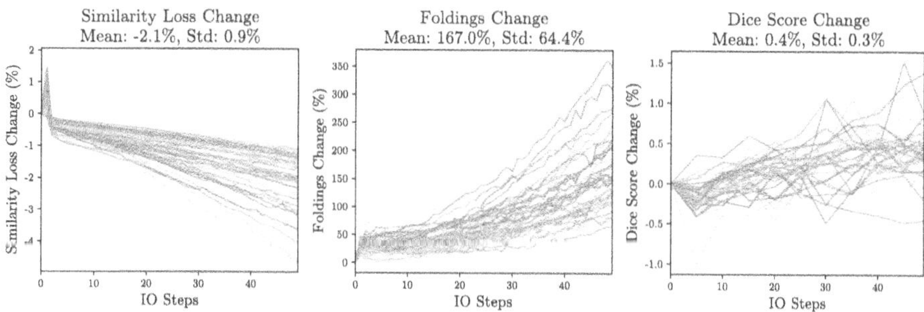

Fig. 2. Dynamics of instance optimization on the 10-class validation subset with VFA-Brain-ID (1K). Dice score is recorded per 5 steps.

5 Conclusion

We introduced a flexible test-time adaptation framework that repurposes pre-trained mono-modal backbones for robust multi-modal registration through contrast-agnostic transfer and lightweight instance optimization. The approach remains orthogonal to the backbone choice, avoids the prohibitive cost of full fine-tuning, and ranks among the top-performing methods on the Learn2Reg 2025 LUMIR benchmark. Our ablation studies further confirm the benefit of Brain-ID based transfer, multi-level compositional refinement, and moderate pretraining. The results demonstrate that even frozen backbones can be effectively adapted to challenging cross-modality settings as a robust alternative to full network finetuning with the proposed framework.

References

1. Balakrishnan, G., Zhao, A., Sabuncu, M.R., Guttag, J., Dalca, A.V.: VoxelMorph: a learning framework for deformable medical image registration. IEEE Trans. Med. Imag. **38**(8), 1788–1800 (2019)
2. Chen, J., Frey, E.C., He, Y., Segars, W.P., Li, Y., Du, Y.: TransMorph: transformer for unsupervised medical image registration. Med. Image Anal. **82**, 102615 (2022)
3. Chen, J., et al.: Beyond the Lumir challenge: the pathway to foundational registration models. arXiv preprint arXiv:2505.24160 (2025)
4. Dalca, A.V., Balakrishnan, G., Guttag, J., Sabuncu, M.R.: Unsupervised learning of probabilistic diffeomorphic registration for images and surfaces. Med. Image Anal. **57**, 226–236 (2019)
5. De Vos, B.D., Berendsen, F.F., Viergever, M.A., Sokooti, H., Staring, M., Išgum, I.: A deep learning framework for unsupervised affine and deformable image registration. Med. Image Anal. **52**, 128–143 (2019)
6. Demir, B., et al.: MultiGradICON: a foundation model for multimodal medical image registration. In: International Workshop on Biomedical Image Registration, pp. 3–18. Springer (2024)
7. Dufumier, B., Grigis, A., Victor, J., Ambroise, C., Frouin, V., Duchesnay, E.: OpenBHB: a large-scale multi-site brain MRI data-set for age prediction and debiasing. Neuroimage **263**, 119637 (2022)
8. van Harten, L., Van Herten, R.L.M., Stoker, J., Isgum, I.: Deformable image registration with geometry-informed implicit neural representations. In: Medical Imaging with Deep Learning (2023)
9. Heinrich, M.P., et al.: MIND: modality independent neighbourhood descriptor for multi-modal deformable registration. Med. Image Anal. **16**(7), 1423–1435 (2012)
10. Hoffmann, M., Billot, B., Greve, D.N., Iglesias, J.E., Fischl, B., Dalca, A.V.: SynthMorph: learning contrast-invariant registration without acquired images. IEEE Trans. Med. Imaging **41**(3), 543–558 (2021)
11. Iglesias, J.E., et al.: SynthSR: a public AI tool to turn heterogeneous clinical brain scans into high-resolution T1-weighted images for 3D morphometry. Sci. Adv. **9**(5), eadd3607 (2023)
12. King, A.P., et al.: Registering preprocedure volumetric images with intraprocedure 3-d ultrasound using an ultrasound imaging model. IEEE Trans. Med. Imag. **29**(3), 924–937 (2010)
13. Klein, S., Staring, M., Pluim, J.P.: Evaluation of optimization methods for nonrigid medical image registration using mutual information and b-splines. IEEE Trans. Imag. Proc. **16**(12), 2879–2890 (2007)
14. Liu, P., Puonti, O., Hu, X., Alexander, D.C., Iglesias, J.E.: Brain-ID: learning contrast-agnostic anatomical representations for brain imaging. In: European Conference on Computer Vision, pp. 322–340. Springer (2024)
15. Liu, Y., Chen, J., Wei, S., Carass, A., Prince, J.: On finite difference Jacobian computation in deformable image registration. Int. J. Comput. Vis., 1–11 (2024)
16. Liu, Y., Chen, J., Zuo, L., Carass, A., Prince, J.L.: Vector field attention for deformable image registration. J. Med. Imag. **11**(6), 064001–064001 (2024)
17. Marcus, D.S., Wang, T.H., Parker, J., Csernansky, J.G., Morris, J.C., Buckner, R.L.: Open Access Series of Imaging Studies (OASIS): cross-sectional MRI data in young, middle aged, nondemented, and demented older adults. J. Cogn. Neurosci. **19**(9), 1498–1507 (2007)

18. Mok, T.C., et al.: Modality-agnostic structural image representation learning for deformable multi-modality medical image registration. In: Proceedings of the IEEE/CVF Conference on Computer Vision and Pattern Recognition, pp. 11215–11225 (2024)
19. Mok, T.C., et al.: Deformable medical image registration under distribution shifts with neural instance optimization. In: International Workshop on Machine Learning in Medical Imaging, pp. 126–136. Springer (2023)
20. Niethammer, M., Kwitt, R., Vialard, F.X.: Metric learning for image registration. In: Proceedings of the IEEE/CVF Conference on Computer Vision and Pattern Recognition, pp. 8463–8472 (2019)
21. Qin, C., Shi, B., Liao, R., Mansi, T., Rueckert, D., Kamen, A.: Unsupervised deformable registration for multi-modal images via disentangled representations. In: Chung, A.C.S., Gee, J.C., Yushkevich, P.A., Bao, S. (eds.) IPMI 2019. LNCS, vol. 11492, pp. 249–261. Springer, Cham (2019). https://doi.org/10.1007/978-3-030-20351-1_19
22. Ronneberger, O., Fischer, P., Brox, T.: U-Net: convolutional networks for biomedical image segmentation. In: Navab, N., Hornegger, J., Wells, W.M., Frangi, A.F. (eds.) MICCAI 2015, Part III. LNCS, vol. 9351, pp. 234–241. Springer, Cham (2015). https://doi.org/10.1007/978-3-319-24574-4_28
23. Rueckert, D., Schnabel, J.A.: Model-based and data-driven strategies in medical image computing. Proc. IEEE **108**(1), 110–124 (2019)
24. Siebert, H., Großbröhmer, C., Hansen, L., Heinrich, M.P.: ConvexAdam: self-configuring dual-optimisation-based 3d multitask medical image registration. IEEE Trans. Med. Imag. (2024)
25. Sotiras, A., Davatzikos, C., Paragios, N.: Deformable medical image registration: a survey. IEEE Trans. Med. Imag. **32**(7), 1153–1190 (2013)
26. Staring, M., van der Heide, U.A., Klein, S., Viergever, M.A., Pluim, J.P.: Registration of cervical MRI using multifeature mutual information. IEEE Trans. Med. Imag. **28**(9), 1412–1421 (2009)
27. Taha, A., Chevalier, R., et al.: Magnetic resonance imaging datasets with anatomical fiducials for quality control and registration. Sci. Data **10**(1), 449 (2023)
28. Tian, L., et al.: uniGradICON: a foundation model for medical image registration. arXiv preprint arXiv:2403.05780 (2024)
29. de Vos, B.D., van der Velden, B.H., Sander, J., Gilhuijs, K.G., Staring, M., Išgum, I.: Mutual information for unsupervised deep learning image registration. In: Medical Imaging 2020: Image Processing, vol. 11313, pp. 155–161. SPIE (2020)
30. Wolterink, J.M., Zwienenberg, J.C., Brune, C.: Implicit neural representations for deformable image registration. In: Medical Imaging with Deep Learning, pp. 1349–1359. PMLR (2022)
31. Zhang, Y., Zhao, Y., Tao, Q.: Bridging classical and learning-based iterative registration through deep equilibrium models. arXiv preprint arXiv:2507.00582 (2025)

Generalizable Learning-Based Image Registration via Self-supervised Multi-modal Representation Learning from Single-Modal Data

Chih-Ping Chen(✉), Chi-Hsuan Tsao, and Chien-Yao Wang

Institute of Information Science, Academia Sinica, Taipei, Taiwan
{genephil,salamancatsao,kinyiu}@iis.sinica.edu.tw

Abstract. Neurological disorders of the brain, including trauma, inflammation, and tumors often have complex etiologies and can affect cognition. Magnetic Resonance Imaging (MRI) is crucial for diagnosing brain diseases, with multimodal scans and varying field strengths providing complementary information. Accurate registration in heterogeneous images enhances interpretability and clinical utility. Current methods often struggle with cross-field-strength, cross-dataset, and cross-modality alignment. We propose an unsupervised registration framework that leverages Shuffle Remap to simulate diverse modalities and employs self-supervised image-to-image and latent-to-latent translation tasks for improved feature alignment. Evaluated in the Learn2Reg LUMIR 2025 Challenge validation set under zero-shot scenarios, our method achieves a Dice score of 75.73%, demonstrating strong generalization and robustness in heterogeneous MRI registration.

Keywords: Image registration · Self-supervised learning · Magnetic resonance imaging

1 Introduction

Medical image registration is a fundamental step in medical image analysis [5], enabling the alignment of images from different sources, time points, patients, or imaging modalities to accurately monitor disease progression [18,21]. Effective registration of structural information across varying magnetic field strengths, pathological brain lesions, image contrasts, or modalities (e.g., MRI-T1 vs. MRI-T2, MRI vs. PET, MRI vs. CT) is critical for integrative analyses and longitudinal monitoring [1,6]. However, images acquired under diverse conditions—such as different scanning techniques, resolutions, and intensity distributions—pose significant challenges for conventional registration methods, which often fail to deliver stable and accurate results [17].

With the advent of deep learning, VoxelMorph proposed by Balakrishnan et al. [2] has emerged as a leading learning-based registration model. Leveraging a

J. Chen et al. (Eds.): Learn2Reg 2025, LNCS 16254, pp. 62–70, 2026.
https://doi.org/10.1007/978-3-032-25169-5_8

U-Net architecture, it demonstrates strong performance in same-modality scenarios [16]. Yet, differences in modality, contrast, and acquisition protocols limit the effectiveness of traditional similarity metrics, reducing alignment accuracy in critical anatomical regions [10].

In the LUMIR 2025 Challenge [4,8,19], our goal is to evaluate the generalization capability of registration models under an unsupervised learning framework, focusing particularly on zero-shot tasks. The challenge assesses model robustness under domain shifts, including variations in imaging modality, magnetic field strength, and pathological changes. The training dataset consists of T1-weighted MRI scans from 3,384 subjects across 10 public sources, preprocessed to $160 \times 224 \times 192$ voxels with $1 \times 1 \times 1$ mm isotropic resolution. Validation uses 40 subjects, including 10 healthy individuals from the training distribution, 10 healthy controls from external datasets, 10 high-field MRI scans, and 10 multi-modal images for T1-to-T2 registration. The final testing set comprises over 1,590 zero-shot images, encompassing challenging scenarios such as high-field MRI, pathological brains, and alternate MRI contrasts, serving as a comprehensive benchmark for evaluating model generalization.

This work presents a novel unsupervised learning method for multi-modal medical image registration using single-modal data. The approach leverages Shuffle Remap [13] to simulate diverse imaging modalities and incorporates image-to-image and latent-to-latent self-supervised translation tasks to learn robust correspondences across modalities, magnetic field strengths, and pathological variations. The framework is flexible and can be integrated with existing registration models to further improve performance. On the validation leaderboard, it achieves a Dice score of 75.73%, demonstrating strong generalization and robustness in multi-modal MRI registration.

2 Methods

2.1 Overview

We propose a registration framework trained via a two-stage scheme. To foster a highly generalizable feature representation, the training process leverages a multi-task self-supervised learning approach, as illustrated in Fig. 1. This process is driven by two components: (1) extensive data augmentation (e.g., Shuffle Remap [13] and intensity transformations to improve performance across diverse imaging conditions, and (2) the proposed self-supervised auxiliary (SSL) tasks—image-to-image (I2I) and latent-to-latent (L2L) translation—designed to facilitate the learning of modality-invariant features.

The first stage of the training curriculum optimizes for registration accuracy, while the second stage incorporates an NDV loss [15] to regularize the deformation fields for smoothness and physical plausibility. During inference, the predicted deformation field for each image pair undergoes instance optimization (25 steps) without the use of SSL tasks, improving the framework's robustness and adaptability to unseen domains.

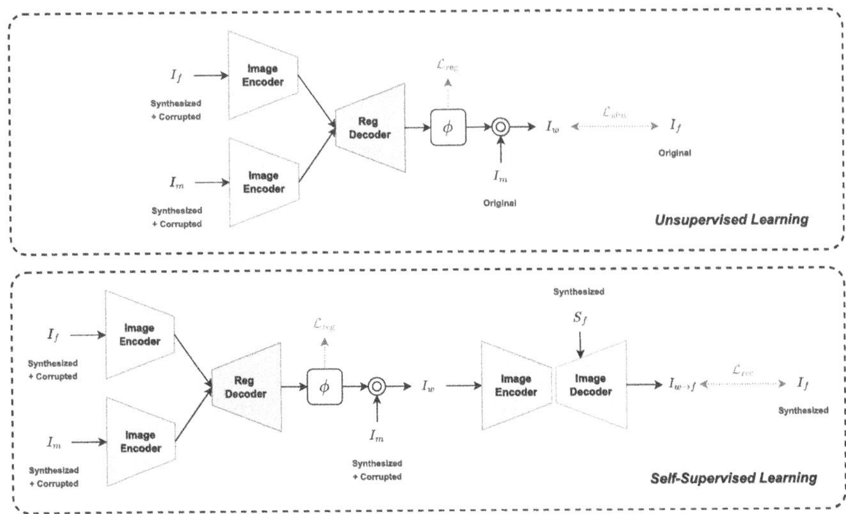

Fig. 1. Self-Supervised Image Registration Framework. Our self-supervised image registration framework learns modality-invariant and generalizable features through a multi-task approach. The network takes a *synthesized + corrupted* movingfixed image pair (augmented with Shuffle Remap and intensity transformations) as input. An unsupervised similarity loss, computed between the warped *original* moving image and the *original* fixed image, drives deformation field prediction for alignment. An auxiliary self-supervised loss enhances features through a shared-parameter modality transfer model, which transforms the warped *synthesized + corrupted* image into the appearance of the fixed *synthesized* image.

2.2 Data Augmentation

Our data augmentation strategy, designed to improve generalization, combines both offline and online components. The primary component, Shuffle Remap, simulates novel modalities. Prior to training, we perform an offline synthesis step: for each original training image, we generate a corresponding pool of 32 synthesized versions by applying 32 distinct parameter sets. Each set defines all parameters required by the Shuffle Remap algorithm, including the number of intensity ranges (varying from 2 to 8).

During each training iteration, the online augmentation pipeline proceeds in two steps. First, with a 50% probability, the original input image is stochastically replaced with a random sample from its synthesized pool. Second, a composite intensity transformation is applied to the resulting image with a 50% probability, comprising a series of MRI-specific augmentations from the MONAI framework [3,7] (*RandBiasField*, *RandKSpaceSpikeNoise*, *RandAdjustContrast*, *RandGaussianSmooth*, *RandGibbsNoise*, *RandGaussianSharpen*, *RandSimulateLowResolution*, and *RandGaussianNoise*). An example illustrating the augmentation process is shown in Fig. 2.

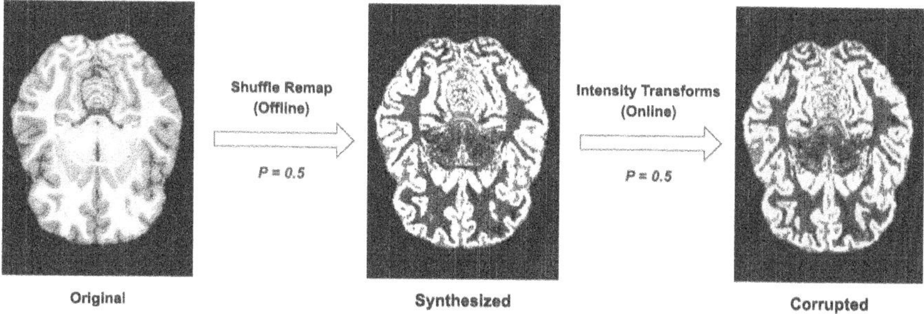

Fig. 2. Data Augmentation. In each training iteration, augmentation is applied in two steps. First, with 50% probability, the original input is replaced by a random Shuffle-Remapped sample to generate a synthesized image [13]. Second, with 50% probability, a composite intensity transformation is applied to produce a corrupted image.

2.3 Self-supervised Multi-modal Representation Learning

We introduce two model-agnostic, self-supervised auxiliary tasks to enhance cross-modality registration (Fig. 3).

The first task, image-to-image (I2I) translation, learns modality correspondences. We first warp the moving image I_m via the predicted deformation field to yield an aligned image I_w. An image decoder, conditioned on the fixed image's modality vector, then reconstructs $I_{w \to f}$. We define a reconstruction loss, $\mathcal{L}_{\text{rec}}$, as the Local Least Squares Error [11] between the reconstructed image $I_{w \to f}$ and the fixed image I_f.

To prevent the I2I synthesis from introducing spatial distortions, the second task, latent-to-latent (L2L) translation, enforces geometric consistency. We first extract multi-scale features from both I_w and I_f. Instance Normalization is then applied to these features. We define an invariance loss, $\mathcal{L}_{\text{inv}}$, as the Mean Squared Error (MSE) between the normalized feature sets.

2.4 Model Architecture

Our architecture is built upon two representative baselines: GroupMorph [20] and SITReg [11]. We replace the native encoders of these baselines with a custom U-Net based encoder for our auxiliary SSL tasks. GroupMorph introduces a grouping-combination strategy, where it predicts and integrates multiple sub-deformation fields to simultaneously capture large-scale and fine-grained transformations. SITReg, in contrast, is an architecture designed to enforce classical properties like symmetry and inverse consistency by construction, utilizing a multi-resolution scheme and a memory-efficient layer for field inversion.

Focusing on the SITReg framework, we systematically investigate several architectural variants. These are based on a standard (*SITReg*) and a large (*SITReg-L*) configuration, to which we apply a series of cumulative enhancements: the -R suffix signifies the incorporation of Residual blocks and Local correlation [14]; the -I suffix adds an Iterative refinement step [12]; and the -F suffix

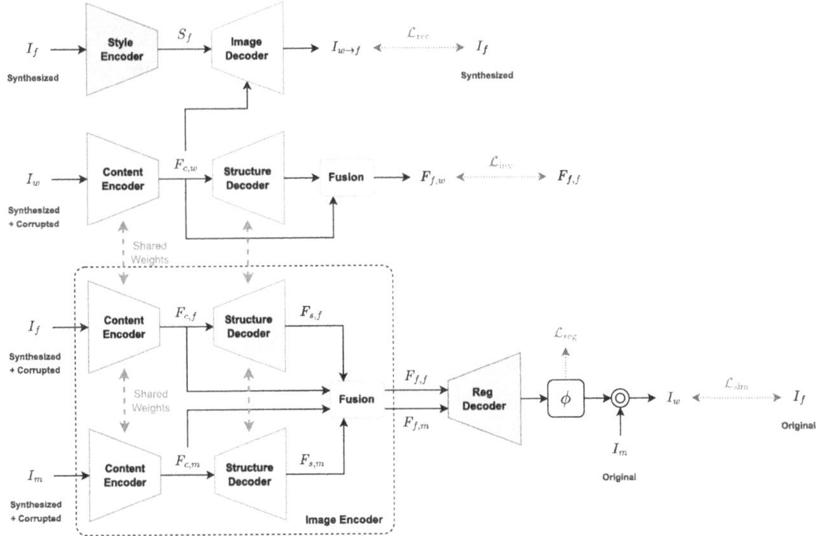

Fig. 3. Self-Supervised Multi-modal Representation Learning. Our self-supervised method jointly optimizes two tasks: (1) Image-to-Image (I2I) translation learns modality correspondences by reconstructing the warped moving image I_w into the fixed modality, with a reconstruction loss $\mathcal{L}_{\text{rec}}$ (Local Least Squares Error [11]) against I_f. (2) Latent-to-Latent (L2L) translation enforces geometric consistency by aligning multi-scale normalized features of I_w and I_f using an invariance loss $\mathcal{L}_{\text{inv}}$ (MSE).

denotes a feature Fusion module that merges features from the Content Encoder and the Structure Decoder, leading to our most advanced models, *SITRegRF-L* and *SITRegRIF-L*.

3 Results

3.1 Training Details

All experiments were conducted on NVIDIA RTX PRO 6000 GPUs. In each epoch, 4000 fixed/moving image pairs were randomly sampled for model training. We employed the same loss function, Loss $= \mathcal{L}_{\text{sim}} + \lambda \cdot \mathcal{L}_{\text{reg}}$, with $1 - \text{NCC}$ as similarity loss and diffusion as smoothness regularization. λ was empirically set to 1.

3.2 Ablation Study

We conduct a series of ablation studies to validate our proposed pipeline, with our development process illustrated in Fig. 4 and quantitative results in Table 1. Our final validated method, built upon the SITRegRF-L baseline, achieves a

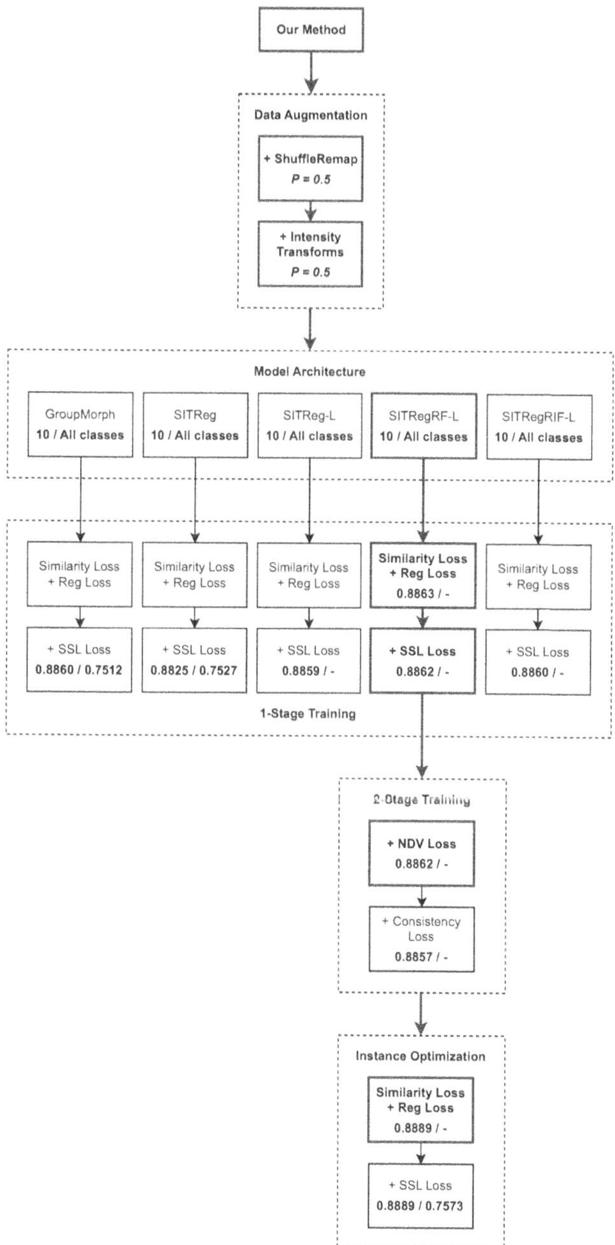

Fig. 4. Development Process. The figure summarizes the five-stage development process for the LUMIR 2025 Challenge: Data Augmentation, Model Architecture, First-Stage Training, Second-Stage Training, and Instance Optimization. Numbers below each block show Dice scores for 10 all classes on the validation set, and blue blocks highlight the final design adopted in our method. (Color figure online)

Table 1. Ablation study of different stages in the development process for the LUMIR 2025 Challenge on the validation set.

	Dice↑		HD95↓	MM Dice↑	NDV(%)↓
	All classes	10 classes	10 classes	10 classes	
Model Architecture					
GroupMorph	0.7512	0.8860	2.6122	**0.8770**	0.06068
SITReg	0.7527	0.8825	2.6315	0.8741	0.00009
SITReg-L	–	0.8859	2.5832	0.8758	**0.00005**
SITRegRF-L	–	**0.8862**	2.5689	0.8760	0.00008
SITRegRIF-L	–	0.8860	**2.5263**	0.8764	0.00018
First-Stage Training					
w/o SSL	–	**0.8863**	**2.5375**	0.8745	0.00012
w/ SSL	–	0.8862	2.5689	**0.8760**	**0.00008**
Second-Stage Training					
w/o Consistency Loss	–	**0.8862**	**2.5720**	**0.8759**	0.0
w/ Consistency Loss	–	0.8857	2.5735	0.8757	0.0
Instance Optimization					
w/o SSL	–	**0.8889**	**2.5289**	**0.8801**	0.0
w/ SSL	0.7573	0.8889	2.5341	0.8801	0.0

peak 10-class Dice score of 0.8889 on the LUMIR 2025 Challenge validation set. The following analysis justifies the selection of our baseline architecture and each component of our training and inference strategy.

Model Architecture. We begin by selecting a strong baseline from several representative architectures. As reported in Table 1, SITRegRF-L achieves the highest Dice score (0.8862) and is thus selected as the foundation for our experiments.

First-Stage Training. Despite a marginal effect on primary Dice and HD95 metrics, we incorporate Self-Supervised Learning (SSL) for its crucial role in learning modality-invariant features, as evidenced by a significant improvement in Multi-Modal (MM) Dice (0.8760 vs. 0.8745).

Second-Stage Training. Including an additional group consistency loss [9,14] degraded performance on both Dice (0.8862 to 0.8857) and HD95 (2.5720 to 2.5735); we therefore exclude it from our final pipeline.

Instance Optimization. The final instance optimization process provides a substantial performance boost, increasing the Dice score from 0.8862 to its peak of 0.8889. We perform this optimization without SSL, as this improves HD95 (2.5289 vs. 2.5341) while maintaining the top Dice score.

3.3 Leaderboard Performance

Our method achieved an overall Dice score of 75.73% on the leaderboard, demonstrating strong performance across all metrics. The results include a TRE of 2.2651, an HD95 of 3.2182, an NDV of 0.0043%, and competitive Dice scores of 77.54% (in-domain), 76.01% (out-of-domain), and 73.65% (multi-modal). These findings indicate our method's strong generalizability, even in challenging zero-shot testing scenarios.

4 Discussion

In this work, we addressed the challenge of robust unsupervised brain MRI registration across cross-dataset, cross-modality, and cross-field-strength variations. By introducing Shuffle Remap for modality simulation and employing self-supervised image-to-image and latent-to-latent translation tasks, our method effectively learns cross-domain correspondences and enhances generalization. Evaluation in the LUMIR 2025 Challenge validation set demonstrates competitive performance, achieving a Dice score of 75.73% on the validation set, highlighting its robustness across diverse and unseen scenarios. These findings underscore the promise of combining modality simulation with self-supervised strategies to advance registration in heterogeneous medical imaging.

Acknowledgments. We would like to thank the organizers of the MICCAI 2025 Learn2Reg challenge. This work was supported by the following projects: AS-TP-114-M01, AS-IAIA-114-M05, and NSTC 114-2222-E-001-002-MY3.

References

1. Azam, M.A., Khan, K.B., Ahmad, M., Mazzara, M.: Multimodal medical image registration and fusion for quality enhancement. Comput. Mater. Continua **68**(1), 821–840 (2021)
2. Balakrishnan, G., Zhao, A., Sabuncu, M.R., Guttag, J., Dalca, A.V.: Voxelmorph: a learning framework for deformable medical image registration. IEEE Trans. Med. Imag. **38**(8), 1788–1800 (2019)
3. Cardoso, M.J., et al.: MONAI: an open-source framework for deep learning in healthcare. arXiv preprint arXiv:2211.02701 (2022)
4. Chen, J., et al.: Beyond the LUMIR challenge: the pathway to foundational registration models. arXiv preprint arXiv:2505.24160 (2025)
5. Chen, X., et al.: Recent advances and clinical applications of deep learning in medical image analysis. Med. Image Anal. **79**, 102444 (2022)
6. Darzi, F., Bocklitz, T.: A review of medical image registration for different modalities. Bioengineering **11**(8), 786 (2024)

7. Dey, N., et al.: Learning general-purpose biomedical volume representations using randomized synthesis. arXiv preprint arXiv:2411.02372 (2024)
8. Dufumier, B., Grigis, A., Victor, J., Ambroise, C., Frouin, V., Duchesnay, E.: OpenBHB: a large-scale multi-site brain MRI data-set for age prediction and debiasing. Neuroimage **263**, 119637 (2022)
9. Gu, D., et al.: Pair-wise and group-wise deformation consistency in deep registration network. In: Martel, A.L., et al. (eds.) MICCAI 2020. LNCS, vol. 12263, pp. 171–180. Springer, Cham (2020). https://doi.org/10.1007/978-3-030-59716-0_17
10. Hammoudeh, A., Dupont, S.: Deep learning in medical image registration: introduction and survey. arXiv preprint arXiv:2309.00727 (2023)
11. Honkamaa, J., Marttinen, P.: SITReg: multi-resolution architecture for symmetric, inverse consistent, and topology preserving image registration. Mach. Learn. Biomed. Imaging **2**, 2148–2194 (2024). https://doi.org/10.59275/j.melba.2024-276b, https://melba-journal.org/2024:026
12. Jian, B., Pan, J., Ghahremani, M., Rueckert, D., Wachinger, C., Wiestler, B.: Mamba? catch the hype or rethink what really helps for image registration. In: Modat, M., Simpson, I., Špiclin, Ž., Bastiaansen, W., Hering, A., Mok, T.C.W. (eds.) WBIR 2024. LNCS, vol. 15249, pp. 86–97. Springer, Cham (2024). https://doi.org/10.1007/978-3-031-73480-9_7
13. Kong, L., et al.: Indescribable multi-modal spatial evaluator. In: Proceedings of the IEEE/CVF Conference on Computer Vision and Pattern Recognition, pp. 9853–9862 (2023)
14. Liu, H., Ruan, D., Sheng, K.: Unsupervised deformable image registration revisited: Enhancing performance with registration-specific designs. In: Medical Imaging with Deep Learning-Short Papers (2025)
15. Liu, Y., Chen, J., Wei, S., Carass, A., Prince, J.: On finite difference Jacobian computation in deformable image registration. Int. J. Comput. Vision **132**(9), 3678–3688 (2024)
16. McKinley, R., Rummel, C.: Cortexmorph: Fast cortical thickness estimation via diffeomorphic registration using voxelmorph. In: Greenspan, H., et al. (eds.) MICCAI 2023. LNCS, vol. 14229, pp. 730–739. Springer, Cham (2023). https://doi.org/10.1007/978-3-031-43999-5_69
17. Song, G., Han, J., Zhao, Y., Wang, Z., Du, H.: A review on medical image registration as an optimization problem. Current Med. Imaging **13**(3), 274–283 (2017)
18. Song, X., Xu, X., Zhang, J., Reyes, D.M., Yan, P.: Dino-Reg: efficient multimodal image registration with distilled features. IEEE Trans. Med. Imag. (2025)
19. Taha, A., et al.: Magnetic resonance imaging datasets with anatomical fiducials for quality control and registration. Sci. Data **10**(1), 449 (2023)
20. Tan, Z., Zhang, L., Lv, Y., Ma, Y., Lu, H.: GroupMorph: medical image registration via grouping network with contextual fusion. IEEE Trans. Med. Imag. **43**(11), 3807–3819 (2024). https://doi.org/10.1109/TMI.2024.3400603
21. Zhang, Y., et al.: mmformer: multimodal medical transformer for incomplete multimodal learning of brain tumor segmentation. In: Wang, L., Dou, Q., Fletcher, P.T., Speidel, S., Li, S. (eds.) MICCAI 2022. LNCS, vol. 13435, pp. 107–117. Springer, Cham (2022). https://doi.org/10.1007/978-3-031-16443-9_11

Swin-CNN Hybrid Framework for Enhanced Deformable Image Registration

Lyndon Y. L. Chan(✉) and Albert C. S. Chung

Department of Computer Science and Engineering, The Hong Kong University of Science and Technology, Hong Kong, China
yllchan@connect.ust.hk, achung@cse.ust.hk

Abstract. Deformable image registration is a key process in medical imaging for aligning multiple images captured across different times, subjects, or modalities. While traditional registration algorithms require significant time for iterative optimization, modern deep-learning approaches have demonstrated promising results in both accuracy and efficiency. However, challenges remain in interpretability, and the ability to model realistic continuous deformations for large-scale transformations. Observations from last year's LUMIR challenge reveal that top-performing models often utilize dual-stream encoder designs and coarse-to-fine strategies for deformation estimation. Hence, inspired by these effective design patterns, we introduce SwinCNNReg, a novel end-to-end framework utilizing a Swin Transformer-CNN alternate block encoder coupled with a dual CNN-Transformer decoder. We validate our method against the LUMIR 2025 challenge datasets, including T1-weighted brain MRIs and multi-modal imaging scenarios.

Keywords: Image registration · Medical image challenge · Hybrid Encoder · Dual Decoder

1 Introduction

Deformable image registration aims to align images taken at different times, different subjects, and different modalities accurately by determining the correspondence between their features. This is important for fair comparison, diagnosis, and image-guided surgery in medical image analysis. While current deep learning-based methodologies [1,5,19] achieve high accuracy and efficiency, they often struggle with other challenges. One major challenge is that these approaches are not capable of performing fine-tuning or refinements of the deformation fields. This limitation can result in suboptimal alignment, particularly in scenarios involving substantial anatomical changes or large-scale deformations. Furthermore, these models usually focus solely on either local (via CNNs) or global features (via Transformers).

J. Chen et al. (Eds.): Learn2Reg 2025, LNCS 16254, pp. 71–78, 2026.
https://doi.org/10.1007/978-3-032-25169-5_9

In recent years, there has been an increasing trend in combining Convolutional Neural Networks (CNNs) and Transformers to leverage their complementary strengths in medical image analysis. This trend has led to the development of a hybrid architecture that aims to enhance feature extraction capabilities by utilizing CNNs for local context and Transformers for global context. For instance, the work by Zhang et al. [18] introduces an alternate encoder and dual decoder network that effectively captures both local and global information for medical image segmentation. Similarly, Fang and Wang [8] propose a CNN-transformer-based hierarchical network for medical image registration, showing improved performance by integrating these two powerful paradigms. These advancements highlight the potential of hybrid models to address the inherent limitations of traditional approaches in medical imaging tasks, specifically for tasks that require both a global and a detailed field of view.

In last year's LUMIR challenge [4,7,16], several observations were made among the top-performing entries. Most of these models [10,12,17] had a dual-stream encoder architecture, allowing separate encoders to extract features from moving and fixed images independently. In this setup, the encoder itself focuses on obtaining feature representations from the images, while the decoder is responsible for finding correspondences and estimating the deformation field based on the separately encoded feature maps. Additionally, coarse-to-fine strategies [4,10,12,17] for deformation estimation are widely employed, emphasizing the importance of processing feature maps at different resolutions to capture both local and global deformations. These insights highlight the importance of architectural choices and guide our model development in the balance between local and global features.

This paper will continue to focus on the LUMIR 2025 challenge [4,7,16], which includes a T1-weighted brain MRI dataset from healthy controls while having more demanding validation scenarios. We are required to train our models to achieve high accuracy under standard conditions and demonstrate robustness across zero-shot tasks that involve significant domain shifts, such as from healthy T1 brain MRI to high-field MRI or pathological brain imaging. Benchmarks will include multi-modal registration tasks, providing a comprehensive assessment of model generalizability across diverse neuroimaging applications.

In response to the problems identified above, we propose SwinCNNReg, an end-to-end deep learning model that integrates an alternate Swin Transformer-CNN encoder [8,18] with a dual CNN-Transformer decoder. Unlike previous works that employ either a Laplacian pyramid framework [13,14] or a single coarse-to-fine decoder [10,12,17], SwinCNNReg uniquely leverages a dual decoder with dedicated CNN and Transformer pathways. The hybrid encoder extracts both fine-grained local features and long-range spatial dependencies, which are then processed separately by our dual decoder, and dynamically fused using a gated feature fusion block [15] at each level, ensuring global structural consistency and local precision.

To enhance generalization and specifically address the challenge's zero-shot tasks, we employ SynthSR [2,3,11] to synthesize standardized input images from the diverse validation and testing datasets during inference. This preprocessing step helps mitigate domain shift, enabling a single model to handle contrasting MRI protocols and the presence of pathologies robustly.

2 Method

For deformable image registration, the resulting deformation field ϕ serves to align the moving image M, to be close to the fixed image F, ensuring a coherent representation of shared anatomical structures. Deep learning approaches typically frame this challenge as a learning task $\phi = f_\theta(F, M)$ [6,9]. Most of them [1,5,19] focus on predicting the deformation field directly from the input images, employing a discriminative approach. Unlike them, our approach, SwinCNNReg, incorporates a hybrid Swin Transformer-CNN architecture to predict the deformation field from both local and global contexts of the images.

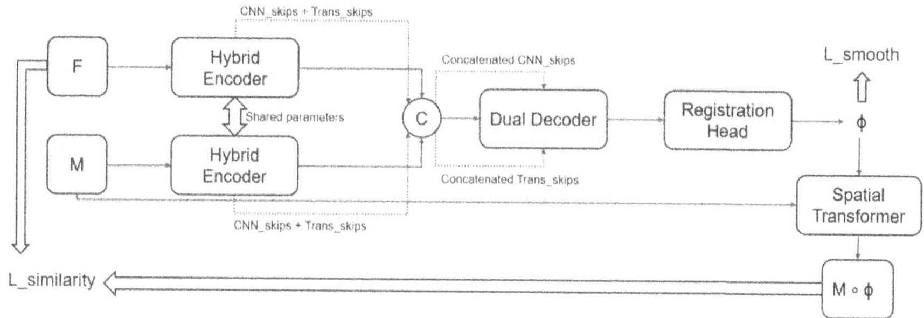

Fig. 1. Architecture of the proposed SwinCNNReg. The model takes a Moving image (**M**) and a Fixed image (**F**) as input. Each image is encoded by a dedicated Hybrid Encoder. The extracted feature maps are then concatenated (C) and processed by a Dual Decoder. The dotted arrows represent the skip connections, which are also concatenated together with features from cnn and transformer respectively in each layer. The Registration Head predicts a dense deformation field ϕ, which is then used by a Spatial Transformer to warp the moving image, producing the final output $\mathbf{M} \circ \phi$.

2.1 Model Architecture

In this work, we adopt an alternate Swin Transformer-CNN encoder, inspired by the architecture proposed in [18]. This encoder is shared and designed to effectively capture both local and global features from the moving image and fixed image individually, which is essential for accurate deformable image registration. The architecture begins with a patch embedding layer that segments the input images into smaller patches, facilitating efficient processing of high-resolution data. It alternates between convolutional neural network (CNN) stages and Swin Transformer stages. The CNN stages employ residual blocks that progressively downsample the input while increasing feature dimensions, allowing for the extraction of fine details. In contrast, the transformer stages utilize self-attention mechanisms to model global contexts, capturing complex interdependencies among features (Fig. 2).

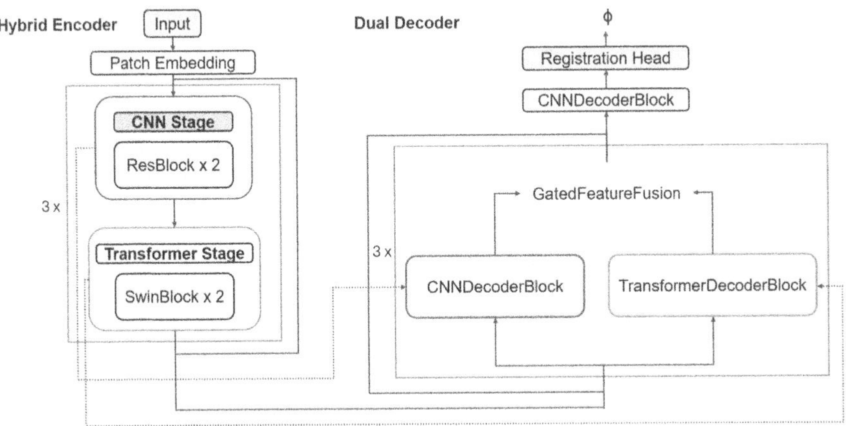

Fig. 2. Overview of the Hybrid Encoder and Dual Decoder. For conciseness, only one encoder is shown here; however, in practice, there is an encoder for each image (fixed and moving images), with their outputs and skip connection maps concatenated, as shown in Fig. 1.

The encoder is focused on feature extraction, while the decoder is responsible for establishing correspondences between the corresponding feature maps and obtaining the deformation field. Before entering the decoder, the feature maps from the moving and fixed images are concatenated. Then, we implement a dual decoder architecture that seperately handles local and global features. The CNN decoder emphasizes the extraction of intricate details, while the Transformer decoder utilizes self-attention mechanisms to capture broader contextual relationships.

To further enhance feature representation, we incorporate gated feature fusion blocks [15], which are designed to merge the output of both the CNN decoder and the Transformer decoder within the decoder stages, ensuring that essential information is retained effectively and optimally combined. The gating mechanism computes a gating mask, G_{local}, which controls the fusion of local and global features. The adaptive fusion process can be expressed mathematically as:

$$F_{\text{refined}} = \alpha \cdot (G_{\text{local}} \odot F_{\text{local}}) + F_{\text{global}}$$

where α is a learnable parameter that scales the contribution of the local features, G_{local} is the gating mask derived from the concatenated feature maps, F_{local} represents the features from the CNN decoder, and F_{global} represents the features from the Transformer decoder. This approach allows our model to adaptively fuse features, leveraging both local details and global context.

Moreover, skip connections are utilized to preserve the output from each encoder block to both the CNN and the Transformer decoder blocks at the same resolution level. This enables the model to look at multi-scale features, thus enhancing the robustness of the deformation field predictions. Overall, this comprehensive framework strikes a balance between local and global feature extraction.

2.2 Training Objective

Our goal is to find an optimal and physically plausible displacement field. Therefore, our loss function for image registration consists of a similarity loss and a regularization loss:

$$L = L_{\text{similarity}} + \lambda L_{\text{smooth}}$$

where λ is the hyperparameter that controls the balance between the two losses, which may be in conflict.

In this paper, we chose to use normalized cross-correlation (NCC) as our similarity measure, which quantifies the similarity between the moving and fixed images. To adapt NCC for minimization in our deep learning model, we define our similarity loss, $L_{\text{similarity}}$, as the negative of the NCC value, allowing the optimization process to focus on maximizing similarity. The regularization loss, L_{smooth}, encourages spatial continuity in the predicted displacement field. By computing differences between neighboring pixels, it prevent any abrupt changes in our field that could lead to unrealistic deformations.

2.3 Implementation Details

Our proposed method is implemented using PyTorch 2.5.1 and runs on an A100 PCIe machine with an AMD Ryzen Threadripper PRO 5955WX 16-core CPU. The model is set to train for 300 epochs, where each epoch consists of 1000 randomly sampled image pairs from the training dataset, with batch size being 1 for computational efficiency. We also use the AdamW optimizer with an initial learning rate of 1×10^{-4} (scheduled via cosine annealing) and a weight decay of 0.01. The loss weighting parameter λ is set to 0.5.

The training dataset provided by the challenge is split with a validation ratio of 0.05 for hyperparameter tuning. We implement early stopping with a patience of 20 epochs based on the validation loss to prevent overfitting.

3 Results

In this section, we are going to validate our model on the LUMIR 2025 challenge [4], which focuses on the registration of large-scale unsupervised brain magnetic resonance images and zero-shot validation.

3.1 Data and Preprocessing

The dataset provided [7,16] contains T1-weighted brain MRI scans sourced from the OpenBHB dataset and multiple publicly available datasets. The training set comprises 3,384 subjects, while the validation set includes 40 subjects divided into four distinct subgroups to facilitate evaluation across varying conditions.

To prepare the MRI scans for analysis, several standard preprocessing steps have been implemented, including skull stripping to eliminate non-brain tissues, affine spatial normalization to align the images, and intensity normalization to standardize the range of voxel intensities. Each MRI scan has also been resampled to ensure isotropic voxel sizes and uniformly cropped to $160 \times 224 \times 192$ voxels by the organizers.

3.2 Inference

During the inference stage, when the pairs of images are from multiple modalities, we employ SynthSR [2], a pre-trained model, to synthesize standardized input images from various validation and testing datasets. This step is important for addressing the challenge's zero-shot tasks, as it helps mitigate domain shifts that may arise from varying MRI protocols and the presence of pathologies. By generating uniform input images from the unseen datasets, this ensures that our model can adapt to contrasting imaging conditions with consistent accuracy, leading to more reliable performance across different validation scenarios.

Furthermore, we observe that the performance improves when a simple binary mask is applied to the synthesized images to filter out the noise and keep important high-frequency features. This mask is generated by identifying valid regions, removing artifacts in the synthesized images from areas with zero intensities in the original images. As a result, it ensures that they focus only on meaningful data.

3.3 Validation Results

Table 1 provides a comprehensive summary of the results of our best model submitted on the validation leaderboard and the results of our current model submitted. We present each metric with its mean and standard deviation, offering insights into the performance and variability of our approach.

Table 1. Validation Results Summary

	DSC ↑	HD95 ↓	TRE_lm ↓	ID_dice ↑	MM_dice ↑	OOD_dice ↑	NDV ↓
Mean	0.7122	3.7365	2.6809	0.7299	0.7039	0.7028	0.2404
Std. Dev.	0.0241	0.4600	0.2585	0.0131	0.0242	0.0228	0.0761
Mean	0.6996	3.8369	2.7938	0.7236	0.6814	0.6937	0.7914
Std. Dev.	0.0267	0.4359	0.3926	0.0117	0.0237	0.0224	0.1661

In image registration, DSC (Dice Similarity Coefficient) measures the overlap between the warped moving segmentation maps and the fixed segmentation maps. HD95 (Hausdorff Distance at 95th Percentile) indicates the maximum distance between the warped moving image and the fixed image boundaries, focusing on the furthest points, while TRE_lm (Target Registration Error in Landmark) tells the distance between landmark points in the warped moving image and the fixed image.

Our model achieves a mean DSC of 0.7122, and a relatively low standard deviation of 0.0241 across different validation samples. The mean HD95 of 3.7365 and mean TRE_lm of 2.6809 also shows a manageable maximum distance between boundaries and landmarks.

4 Discussion

However, as shown in Table 1, there remains significant room for improvement. Further enhancements are necessary. For instance, our model still struggle with extreme anatomical variations, leading to suboptimal accuracy.

The next step would be to examine and test different alternative model architectures. For example, replacing the Swin Transformer with a Vision Transformer might be beneficial, as it is specifically designed to capture global attention across the entire image. In contrast, the Swin Transformer employs a hierarchical approach that balances global and local attention while being fine-tuned for computational efficiency. Moreover, adding a progressive refinement strategy might also be beneficial for the model to perform image registration with subpixel accuracy.

Future work will focus on these enhancements and the implementation of more comprehensive validation strategies to ensure our model's adaptability across diverse imaging scenarios.

References

1. Balakrishnan, G., Zhao, A., Sabuncu, M.R., Guttag, J., Dalca, A.V.: VoxelMorph: a learning framework for deformable medical image registration. IEEE Trans. Med. Imag. **38**(8), 1788–1800 (2019). https://doi.org/10.1109/TMI.2019.2897538
2. Billot, B., et al.: SynthSeg: domain randomisation for segmentation of brain MRI scans of any contrast and resolution. arXiv:2107.09559 [cs] (2021)
3. Billot, B., et al.: SynthSeg: segmentation of brain MRI scans of any contrast and resolution without retraining. Med. Image Anal. **86**, 102789 (2023). https://doi.org/10.1016/j.media.2023.102789
4. Chen, J., et al.: Beyond the LUMIR challenge: the pathway to foundational registration models. arXiv preprint (2025)
5. Chen, J., Frey, E.C., He, Y., Segars, W.P., Li, Y., Du, Y.: TransMorph: transformer for unsupervised medical image registration. Med. Image Anal. **82**, 102615 (2022). https://doi.org/10.1016/j.media.2022.102615
6. Chen, J., et al.: A survey on deep learning in medical image registration: new technologies, uncertainty, evaluation metrics, and beyond. Med. Image Anal. **100**, 103385 (2025). https://doi.org/10.1016/j.media.2024.103385

7. Dufumier, B., et al.: OpenBHB: a large-scale multi-site brain MRI data-set for age prediction and debiasing. Neuroimage **263**, 119637 (2022)
8. Fang, B., Wang, L.: A CNN-transformer-based unsupervised aware hierarchical network for medical image registration. Electron. Lett. **60** (2024). https://doi.org/10.1049/ell2.70124
9. Haskins, G., Kruger, U., Yan, P.: Deep learning in medical image registration: a survey. Mach. Vis. Appl. **31**(8) (2020). https://doi.org/10.1007/s00138-020-01060-x
10. Honkamaa, J., Marttinen, P.: SITReg: multi-resolution architecture for symmetric, inverse consistent, and topology preserving image registration using deformation inversion layers (2024). https://openreview.net/forum?id=gfh8ZbSlyf
11. Iglesias, J.E., et al.: Joint super-resolution and synthesis of 1 mm isotropic MP-RAGE volumes from clinical MRI exams with scans of different orientation, resolution and contrast. NeuroImage **237** (2021)
12. Jian, B., Pan, J., Ghahremani, M., Rueckert, D., Wachinger, C., Wiestler, B.: Mamba? catch the hype or rethink what really helps for image registration. In: Modat, M., Simpson, I., Špiclin, Ž, Bastiaansen, W., Hering, A., Mok, T.C.W. (eds.) WBIR 2024. LNCS, vol. 15249, pp. 86–97. Springer, Cham (2024). https://doi.org/10.1007/978-3-031-73480-9_7
13. Mok, T.C.W., Chung, A.C.S.: Large deformation diffeomorphic image registration with Laplacian pyramid networks. In: Martel, A.L., et al. (eds.) MICCAI 2020. LNCS, vol. 12263, pp. 211–221. Springer, Cham (2020). https://doi.org/10.1007/978-3-030-59716-0_21
14. Mok, T.C.W., Chung, A.C.S.: Conditional deformable image registration with convolutional neural network. In: de Bruijne, M., et al. (eds.) MICCAI 2021. LNCS, vol. 12904, pp. 35–45. Springer, Cham (2021). https://doi.org/10.1007/978-3-030-87202-1_4
15. Qin, J., Xiong, J., Liang, Z.: CNN-transformer gated fusion network for medical image super-resolution. Sci. Rep. **15**, 15338 (2025). https://doi.org/10.1038/s41598-025-00119-x
16. Taha, A., et al.: Magnetic resonance imaging datasets with anatomical fiducials for quality control and registration. Sci. Data **10**(1), 449 (2023)
17. Tan, Z., Zhang, L., Lv, Y., Ma, Y., Lu, H.: GroupMorph: medical image registration via grouping network with contextual fusion. IEEE Trans. Med. Imag. **43**(11), 3807–3819 (2024). https://doi.org/10.1109/TMI.2024.3400603
18. Zhang, L., Guo, X., Sun, H., et al.: Alternate encoder and dual decoder CNN-transformer networks for medical image segmentation. Sci. Reports **15**(8883) (2025). https://doi.org/10.1038/s41598-025-93353-2
19. Zhao, S., Lau, T., Luo, J., Chang, E.I.C., Xu, Y.: Unsupervised 3D end-to-end medical image registration with volume Tweening network. IEEE J. Biomed. Health Inform. **24**(5), 1394–1404 (2020). https://doi.org/10.1109/JBHI.2019.2951024

Efficient Unsupervised Multimodal Brain MR Image Registration with Encoder-Only Network

Xinyao Yu[1(✉)], Yue He[2], Yuxi Zhang[2], Jiazheng Wang[2], Xiang Chen[2], Min Liu[2], and Hang Zhang[3]

[1] National University of Singapore, Singapore, Singapore
xinyao.yu@u.nus.edu
[2] Hunan University, Changsha, China
[3] Cornell University, Ithaca, USA

Abstract. Unsupervised brain MR image registration in mono-modal settings has benefited from amortized neural network learning, enabling fast and accurate registration performance. However, clinically common scenarios such as multi-modal and out-of-domain registration remain challenging. To address these issues, we propose a unified encoder-only image registration (EOIR) framework combined with data augmentation and a cross mutual information function (CMIF). Our approach tackles three key challenges: (1) **Efficient training on large cohorts**: EOIR is a sub-1MB-parameter network that can be trained within a day on nearly 4000 subjects while producing diffeomorphic deformations. (2) **Robustness to multi-center and multi-modality data**: We employ public image synthesis tools such as SynthSR and HACA3, together with Bézier curve-based intensity manipulations, to address inter-center and modality variations. (3) **Driving towards global optima**: In addition to the NCC loss, we incorporate CMIF to guide anatomical alignment toward globally optimal solutions. On the validation set, our method outperforms all baselines in anatomical alignment accuracy while producing diffeomorphic deformations.

Keywords: Deformable image registration · Encoder-only image registration · Cross mutual information function · Image synthesis

1 Introduction

Image registration is a core component of many neuroimaging pipelines, underpinning population studies, longitudinal analyses and atlas-based interpretation. In clinical and research settings, brain MRI data are acquired with a wide range of scanners and protocols; differences in pulse sequences, coil setups, resolution and vendor-specific preprocessing lead to large, systematic shifts in image

X. Yu and Y. He—These authors contributed equally.

J. Chen et al. (Eds.): Learn2Reg 2025, LNCS 16254, pp. 79–88, 2026.
https://doi.org/10.1007/978-3-032-25169-5_10

appearance. These acquisition variabilities, manifesting as contrast changes, differing signal-to-noise ratios and nonuniform voxel sampling, complicate the task of aligning anatomy across subjects and sites [7].

Classical variational and optimization-based registration algorithms [1,16,23] provide principled solutions but rely on assumptions such as brightness constancy or smooth intensity correspondences [11]. These hold in mono-modal settings but break under large inter-site or inter-modal variations. Deep learning methods [2,6,21] accelerate inference through amortized optimization [10], yet have limitations: semi-supervised, label-driven strategies may yield high Dice scores but often produce unrealistic deformations, while models trained on a single dataset or modality generalize poorly to new protocols or modalities [12]. Thus, there is a need for structural, contrast-invariant representations that avoid segmentation shortcuts while remaining efficient and robust under domain shift.

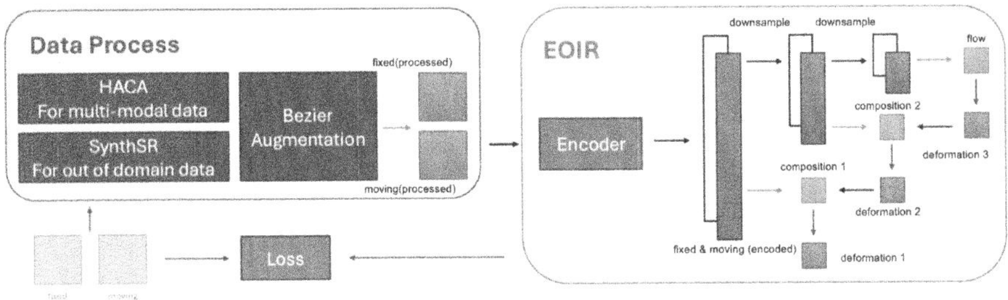

Fig. 1. Overview of the proposed method. The Data Process module includes HACA for multimodal harmonization, SynthSR for reconstruction to a standardized 1 mm isotropic MP-RAGE space, and Bézier-based nonlinear intensity augmentation. The processed fixed and moving images are fed into the EOIR network, which extracts hierarchical features from a Laplacian pyramid and estimates the deformation field. The deformation is applied to the moving image, and the loss is computed using NCC and the proposed CMIF on the original images.

The Learn2Reg 2025 LUMIR task directly addresses this challenge by requiring zero-shot, large-scale brain MRI registration under strict conditions. Methods must be fully unsupervised, trained without segmentation labels or external data, and evaluated on both in-domain accuracy and robustness to out-of-domain and multi-modal scenarios, with containerized execution ensuring reproducibility [4,17]. These requirements promote registration frameworks that generalize across acquisition protocols and modalities while producing smooth, anatomically plausible deformations. To address these challenges, we propose a unified encoder-only image registration (EOIR) framework [5]. It leverages SynthSR [3] and HACA3 [24] for robustness to multi-center and multi-modality data, and applies Bézier curve-based intensity manipulations for data augmentation. Motivated by evidence that alignment accuracy depends on raw-intensity mutual information [12], we further introduce a cross mutual information function (CMIF) loss [20] to guide anatomical alignment toward better optima. On the validation set, our method outperforms all baselines in anatomical alignment accuracy while producing diffeomorphic deformations.

2 Methods

2.1 Efficient Training on Large Cohorts

We adopt the Encoder-Only Image Registration (EOIR) network [5] as the backbone. EOIR is lightweight (< 1M parameters), efficiently trainable, and produces diffeomorphic transformations. It builds on a multi-level Laplacian image pyramid, using three 3D convolution-instance normalization-ReLU blocks (Conv-Blocks) as encoders to extract moving and fixed feature maps, followed by bilinear downsampling. At each pyramid level, the fixed feature map is concatenated with the warped moving feature map from the previous level (if available), passed through three 3D Conv-Blocks for coefficient extraction, and finalized with a linear layer to generate the deformation field (Fig. 1).

2.2 Robustness to Multi-center and Multi-modality Data

Image Harmonization and Synthesis. To mitigate domain shifts from acquisition differences, we integrate the HACA3 harmonization module [24], aligning all training data to a selected high-quality reference image. To address voxel size variations, we employ SynthSR [3], which synthesizes standardized 1 mm isotropic MP-RAGE images from arbitrary scans, improving robustness to resolution, contrast, and orientation differences. We follow the official implementation and use their released weights for harmonization and synthesis.

Bézier Curve for Data Augmentation. To simulate heterogeneous intensity variations across modalities, we adopt a stochastic non-linear intensity augmentation strategy similar to [14]. A Bézier curve defined by random control points $P_i \in [0, 1]^2$ is applied to image intensities:

$$B(t) = \sum_{i=0}^{n} P_i \cdot b_{i,n}(t), \tag{1}$$

where $b_{i,n}(t)$ are Bernstein polynomials. To further enforce contrast-invariant embeddings, we randomly invert the image intensities:

$$I'(x) = \begin{cases} B(I(x)), & p > \delta \\ B(1 - I(x)), & p \leq \delta \end{cases} \quad x \in \Omega, \tag{2}$$

where $p \in [0, 1]$ is a sampled probability and δ is a threshold. This augmentation diversifies training distributions while preserving geometric structures.

Usage. During training, HACA3 and SynthSR are used to harmonize images with varying parameters, and the harmonized copies are stored alongside the originals. At each iteration, either original or harmonized images are randomly loaded, and Bézier curve-based intensity manipulation is applied with 50% probability to both moving and fixed images. Loss computation is always performed on the original images to preserve consistent supervision signals [12]. At inference, HACA3 is applied to multi-modal inputs and SynthSR to out-of-domain inputs for optimal performance.

2.3 Driving Towards Global Optima

In addition to the NCC loss, we incorporate a mutual information loss based on the cross-mutual information function (CMIF) [15,20], which better captures raw-intensity dependencies between moving and fixed images [12]. Given fixed image $I_A \subseteq X_A$ and moving image $I_B \subseteq X_B$, their overlap is denoted as I_{AB}, where $I_{AB} \neq \emptyset$. Each image is first clustered into discrete level sets $A \in \mathbb{Z}$ and $B \in \mathbb{Z}$ using K-means. For each level $a \in A$ and $b \in B$, the marginal and joint histogram entries are computed, from which the marginal and joint Shannon entropies are derived as:

$$H_A = -\sum_{a\in A} \frac{I_A^a \cdot I_B}{N_{AB}} \log \frac{I_A^a \cdot I_B}{N_{AB}}, \tag{3}$$

$$H_B = -\sum_{b\in B} \frac{I_A \cdot I_B^b}{N_{AB}} \log \frac{I_A \cdot I_B^b}{N_{AB}}, \tag{4}$$

$$H_{AB} = -\sum_{a\in A}\sum_{b\in B} \frac{I_A^a \cdot I_B^b}{N_{AB}} \log \frac{I_A^a \cdot I_B^b}{N_{AB}}, \tag{5}$$

where I_A^a and I_B^b denote the binary masks of pixels belonging to cluster levels a and b, respectively, and N_{AB} is the number of overlapping pixels in I_{AB}. The mutual information is then defined as:

$$\mathcal{L}_{\text{CMIF}} = \text{CMIF}(I_A, I_B) = H_A + H_B - H_{AB}. \tag{6}$$

2.4 Overall Loss Composition

For the multi-level image pyramid, we follow the original EOIR design by combining normalized cross-correlation (NCC) loss with a diffusive regularization term. The total loss is computed as an exponentially decayed weighted sum across pyramid levels:

$$\mathcal{L}_{\text{EOIR}} = \sum_{l=1}^{n} \frac{1}{2^{l-1}} \Big[s\big(d(I_m, l) \circ \phi_l, d(I_f, l)\big) + \lambda r(u_l) \Big], \tag{7}$$

where $s(\cdot,\cdot)$ is the dissimilarity function, $d(\cdot, l)$ the downsampling operator, u_l the displacement field, and $r(u_l) = \|\nabla u_l\|^2$ the smoothness penalty. The final objective combines EOIR pyramid loss with CMIF:

$$\mathcal{L}_{\text{total}} = \mathcal{L}_{\text{EOIR}} + \beta\, \mathcal{L}_{\text{CMIF}}. \tag{8}$$

3 Experiments and Results

3.1 Experimental Setup

All experiments were conducted using PyTorch on a system equipped with an NVIDIA A100 GPU. The EOIR model, HACA3 Module, and SynthSR Module were implemented following their default configurations. For data augmentation, the Bézier Module was applied to each sample with probability $p = 0.5$, using $n = 3$ control points, and the image intensity inversion was applied with probability $\delta = 0.5$. The weight for the mutual information loss was set to $\beta = 1$ throughout all experiments.

3.2 Results

All quantitative results in Table 1 (overall metrics) and Table 2 (subset-wise Dice) come from the validation leaderboard. For compact cross-referencing we refer to each row by its ID in the tables. Overall Dice is shown as mean ± standard deviation (%), TRE and HdDist95 are in nanometres (mm %, i.e. nm), and NDV is shown in per-ten-thousand (‱).

Overall Performance. Table 1 shows that the #5 Unified model achieves the best overall result:

- **Overall Dice:** #5 Unified model yields 75.78% ± 2.50%, the highest mean and a small standard deviation.
- **TRE, HdDist95, and NDV:** #5 Unified model produces TRE = 233.28 nm, HdDist95 = 322.23 nm, NDV = 0.05‱. Compared with optimal values TRE = 232.40 nm, HdDist95 = 310.75 nm, NDV = 0.00‱from across 3 different models, the minor gap is an acceptable trade off for Overall Dice.
- **Baselines:** #3 SynthSR+VFA performs competitively with a Overall Dice = 75.36%, while #2 ConvexAdam-MIND and #4 SynthMorph obtain lower Dice (67.32% and 70.12%, respectively). #1 Zero Displacement baseline confirms the expected low overlap (54.16%).

Subset-Wise Performance. Table 2 breaks down Dice by subset (in-domain, out-of-domain, and multi-modal):

- **In-domain data (IDD):** #5 Unified model attains the highest IDD Dice = 77.75%. Several variants that include harmonization also achieve ~77%.
- **Out-of-domain data (OOD):** #5 Unified model attains OOD Dice = 75.11%. #3 SynthSR+VFA is slightly higher with OODDice = 75.45%, indicating that SynthSR normalization can be effective for some cases.
- **Multi-modal data (MMD):** #5 Unified model and the #6 EOIR + Bezier Curve + CMIF variant both reach MMD Dice = 74.48%, showing that Bezier Curve + CMIF are effective for cross-modal alignment.

Table 1. Validation results on overall metrics. "Overall Dice" is reported as mean ± standard deviation.

ID	Model	Overall Dice↑ (%)	TRE↓ (mm) (%)	HdDist95↓ (%)	NDV↓ (‱)
#1	Zero Displacement	54.16 ± 3.41	435.43	481.66	**0.00**
#2	(Baseline) ConvexAdam - MIND	67.32 ± 2.75	250.80	376.96	0.10
#3	(Baseline) SynthSR + VFA	75.36 ± 2.60	249.56	**310.75**	0.74
#4	(Baseline) SynthMorph	70.12 ± 2.65	260.99	357.71	**0.00**
#5	Unified (full recipe)	**75.78** ± 2.50	233.28	322.23	0.05
#6	EOIR + Bezier Curve + CMIF	75.17 ± 2.88	235.20	338.64	0.05
#7	EOIR + Bezier Curve	72.39 ± 5.65	243.42	344.60	0.05
#8	EOIR + Bezier Curve + SynthSR	73.78 ± 2.32	256.06	330.27	0.01
#9	EOIR + Bezier Curve + HACA3	75.11 ± 2.48	239.55	328.84	0.04
#10	EOIR	59.62±23.67	235.00	507.51	0.04

Table 2. Subset-wise Dice scores for in-domain (IDD), out-of-domain (OOD), and multi-modal (MMD) validation cases (percent).

ID	Model	IDD Dice↑ (%)	OOD Dice↑ (%)	MMD Dice↑ (%)
#1	Zero Displacement	56.68	51.89	53.91
#2	(Baseline) ConvexAdam - MIND	69.98	66.21	65.78
#3	(Baseline) SynthSR + VFA	77.44	**75.45**	73.20
#4	(Baseline) SynthMorph	72.62	68.88	68.88
#5	Unified (full recipe)	**77.75**	75.11	**74.48**
#6	EOIR + Bezier Curve + CMIF	77.60	73.43	74.48
#7	EOIR + Bezier Curve	77.22	75.11	64.83
#8	EOIR + Bezier Curve + SynthSR	75.46	73.63	72.25
#9	EOIR + Bezier Curve + HACA3	77.28	73.88	74.18
#10	EOIR	77.73	74.87	26.27

3.3 Ablation-Style Analysis (component Effects)

We use the available variants in Tables 1 and 2 as ablation proxies to quantify the contribution of individual components. In the following, we report concise, numeric comparisons.

Harmonization (HACA3)

- Compare #7 EOIR + Bezier VS #9 EOIR + Bezier + HACA3: adding HACA3 component to a Bezier-augmented training pipeline increases Overall Dice from 72.39% to 75.11% (+2.72 points); and raises Multi-modal Dice from 64.83% to 74.18% (+9.35 points).
- **Conclusion:** HACA3 is a high-impact component for multi-modal performance; it contributes several absolute percentage points in Dice, especially on the MMD subset.

Synthesis (SynthSR)

- Compare #7 EOIR + Bezier VS #8 EOIR + Bezier + SynthSR: utlilizing SynthSR, Multi-modal Dice improves from 64.83% to 72.25% (+7.42 points); Overall Dice improves from 72.39% to 73.78% (+1.39 points), at the cost of a modest TRE increase by ∼12.6 nm.
- **Conclusion:** synthesis is a strong fallback for multi-modal cases and substantially increases MMD Dice, though it can introduce slight localization degradation.

Augmentation (Bézier Curve)

- Compare #7 EOIR + Bezier Curve VS #10 EOIR: adding Bezier Curve augmentation increases Overall Dice from 59.62% to 72.39% (+12.77 points) and MMD Dice from 26.27% to 64.83% (+38.56 points), and a remarkable decrease in HdDist95.
- **Conclusion:** Bézier augmentation improves zero-shot robustness compared with raw EOIR behavior, and can act complementary to harmonization and synthesis.

Cross-Mutual Information Function (CMIF)

- Compare #6 EOIR + Bezier Curve + CMIF VS #7 EOIR + Bezier Curve: adding CMIF loss yields Multi-modal Dice increasing from 64.83% to 74.48% (+9.65 points) and increases Overall Dice from 72.39% to 75.17 (+2.78 points)
- **Conclusion:** CMIF loss stabilizes multi-modal alignment producing near-unified-level MMD results without harming IDD performance.

4 Discussions and Conclusions

Validation on the LUMIR dataset [4,13] reveals two scenarios where learning-based frameworks substantially outperform iterative methods.

Unsupervised Settings with Large-Scale Datasets. In large-scale brain MRI datasets with relatively simple deformations (e.g., 4000-subject LUMIR), iterative methods [16,18], whether continuous [19], discrete [23], or neural instance optimization, consistently lag behind pure learning-based approaches despite extensive tuning. We attribute this to the regularization term, which not only enforces smoothness but also facilitates displacement signal propagation (message passing) [9,22]. With sufficient data, amortized optimization [12] offers no clear advantage from the dissimilarity metric alone, while the network's regularization effectively exploits contextual information [8] through message passing.

Semi-supervised Settings with Label Supervision. When supervision such as segmentation or keypoints is available, learning-based methods often outperform iterative ones by leveraging contextual information from labels. However, auxiliary losses like segmentation loss may reduce smoothness near mask boundaries, yielding implausible fields and higher NDV values.

In summary, the proposed encoder-only framework achieves the best trade-off between accuracy and robustness on the LUMIR validation set. Data harmonization with SynthSR and HACA3 at inference improves robustness to multi-center and multi-modal data, while training-time synthesis, Bézier-based intensity augmentation, and CMIF loss together yield anatomically plausible deformations across in-domain, out-of-domain, and multi-modal scenarios.

References

1. Avants, B.B., Tustison, N., Song, G., et al.: Advanced normalization tools (ants). Insight J. **2**(365), 1–35 (2009)
2. Balakrishnan, G., Zhao, A., Sabuncu, M.R., Guttag, J., Dalca, A.V.: VoxelMorph: a learning framework for deformable medical image registration. IEEE Trans. Med. Imag. **38**(8), 1788–1800 (2019)
3. Billot, B., et al.: SynthSeg: domain randomisation for segmentation of brain MRI scans of any contrast and resolution. arXiv:2107.09559 [cs] (2021)
4. Chen, J.: Beyond the LUMIR challenge: the pathway to foundational registration models (2025). arXiv:2505.24160 arXiv preprint
5. Chen, X., et al.: Encoder-only image registration. IEEE Trans. Circuits Syst, Video Technol (2026)
6. Chen, X.: Spatially covariant image registration with text prompts. IEEE Trans. Neural Networks Learn. Syst. 1–11 (2024)
7. Dufumier, B., Grigis, A., Victorri, B., et al.: OpenBHB: a large-scale multi-site brain MRI data-set for age prediction and debiasing. Neuroimage **263**, 119637 (2022)

8. Heinrich, M.P.: Closing the Gap Between Deep and Conventional Image Registration Using Probabilistic Dense Displacement Networks. In: Shen, D., Liu, T., Peters, T.M., Staib, L.H., Essert, C., Zhou, S., Yap, P.-T., Khan, A. (eds.) MICCAI 2019. LNCS, vol. 11769, pp. 50–58. Springer, Cham (2019). https://doi.org/10.1007/978-3-030-32226-7_6
9. Heinrich, M.P., Papież, B.W., Schnabel, J.A., Handels, H.: Non-parametric Discrete Registration with Convex Optimisation. In: Ourselin, S., Modat, M. (eds.) WBIR 2014. LNCS, vol. 8545, pp. 51–61. Springer, Cham (2014). https://doi.org/10.1007/978-3-319-08554-8_6
10. Hoopes, A., Hoffmann, M., Fischl, B., Guttag, J., Dalca, A.V.: HyperMorph: Amortized Hyperparameter Learning for Image Registration. In: Feragen, A., Sommer, S., Schnabel, J., Nielsen, M. (eds.) IPMI 2021. LNCS, vol. 12729, pp. 3–17. Springer, Cham (2021). https://doi.org/10.1007/978-3-030-78191-0_1
11. Horn, B.K., Schunck, B.G.: Determining optical flow. Artif. Intell. **17**(1–3), 185–203 (1981)
12. Jena, R., Sethi, D., Chaudhari, P., Gee, J.: Deep learning in medical image registration: Magic or mirage? In: The Thirty-eighth Annual Conference on Neural Information Processing Systems (2024)
13. Liu, Y., Chen, J., Wei, S., Carass, A., Prince, J.: On finite difference Jacobian computation in deformable image registration. Int. J. Comput. Vision **132**(9), 3678–3688 (2024)
14. Mok, T.C.W., et al.: Modality-agnostic structural image representation learning for deformable multi-modality medical image registration (2024). https://arxiv.org/abs/2402.18933
15. Öfverstedt, J., Lindblad, J., Sladoje, N.: Fast computation of mutual information in the frequency domain with applications to global multimodal image alignment. Pattern Recogn. Lett. **159**, 196–203 (2022)
16. Siebert, H., Großbröhmer, C., Hansen, L., Heinrich, M.P.: ConvexAdam: self configuring dual-optimisation-based 3D multitask medical image registration. IEEE Trans. Med, Imag (2024)
17. Taha, A., Betancourt, M., Valabregue, R., et al.: Magnetic resonance imaging datasets with anatomical fiducials for quality control and registration. Sci. Data **10**(1), 449 (2023)
18. Tian, X.: Gaussian primitive optimized deformable retinal image registration, (2025). arXiv:2508.16852 arXiv preprint
19. Vercauteren, T., Pennec, X., Perchant, A., Ayache, N.: Diffeomorphic demons: efficient non-parametric image registration. Neuroimage **45**(1), S61–S72 (2009)
20. Wang, J., et al.: Fidelity-imposed displacement editing for the Learn2Reg 2024 SHG-BF challenge (2025). https://arxiv.org/abs/2410.20812
21. Zhang, H., Chen, X., Hu, R., Liu, D., Li, G., Wang, R.: Memwarp: discontinuity-preserving cardiac registration with memorized anatomical filters. In: Linguraru, M.G., et al. (eds.) MICCAI 2024. LNCS, vol. 15003, pp. 671–681. Springer, Cham (2024).https://doi.org/10.1007/978-3-031-72384-1_63
22. Zhang, H., et al.: Unsupervised deformable image registration with structural non-parametric smoothing. In: Oguz, I., Zhang, S., Metaxas, D.N. (eds.) IPMI 2025. LNCS, vol. 15829, pp. 108–124. Springer, Cham (2025). https://doi.org/10.1007/978-3-031-96628-6_8

23. Zhang, H.: VoxelOpt: voxel-adaptive message passing for discrete optimization in deformable abdominal CT registration. arXiv:2506.19975 arXiv preprint (2025)
24. Zuo, L., et al.: HACA3: a unified approach for multi-site MR image harmonization. Comput. Med. Imaging Graph. **109**, 102285 (2023). https://doi.org/10.1016/j.compmedimag.2023.102285

Author Index

J. Chen et al. (Eds.): Learn2Reg 2025, LNCS 16254, p. 89, 2026.
https://doi.org/10.1007/978-3-032-25169-5

The manufacturer's authorised representative in the EU is Springer Nature Customer Service Centre GmbH, Europaplatz 3, 69115 Heidelberg, Germany. If you have any concerns regarding our products, please contact ProductSafety@springernature.com

Printed and bound by CPI Group (UK) Ltd, Croydon, CR0 4YY
13/07/2026
02164995-0001